# ROBuST
## RCOG Assisted Birth Simulation Training

'A solution to the challenge of reducing maternal and neonatal morbidity and mortality during childbirth is to perfect the art of assisted birth by simulation training. ROBuST addresses this much-needed knowledge in this arena. This well-written book with clear illustrations, tables and clinical pathways is by a team of globally recognised experts who perform, train and research in assisted births and have done so for decades. This is an excellent contribution and must be read and used to provide safe and respectful maternity care.'

Sir Sabaratnam Arulkumaran, PhD DSc FRCS FRCOG
Professor Emeritus of O&G, St George's University of London
Past President RCOG, BMA and FIGO

# ROBuST

## RCOG Assisted Birth Simulation Training

## Course Manual

### Second Edition

Edited by

**George Attilakos**
*University College London Hospitals NHS Foundation Trust*

**Sharon Jordan**
*Southmead Hospital, North Bristol NHS Trust*

**Michele Mohajer**
*Shropshire Women & Children's Centre and the Royal Shrewsbury Hospital, Shrewsbury and Telford Hospital NHS Trust*

**Glen Mola**
*School of Medicine and Health Sciences, University of Papua New Guinea*

**Stephen O'Brien**
*Southmead Hospital, North Bristol NHS Trust*

**Dimitrios Siassakos**
*University College London Hospitals NHS Foundation Trust*

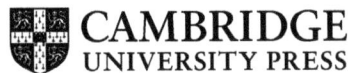
**CAMBRIDGE**
UNIVERSITY PRESS

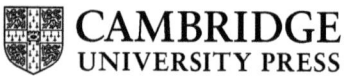

Shaftesbury Road, Cambridge CB2 8EA, United Kingdom

One Liberty Plaza, 20th Floor, New York, NY 10006, USA

477 Williamstown Road, Port Melbourne, VIC 3207, Australia

314–321, 3rd Floor, Plot 3, Splendor Forum, Jasola District Centre, New Delhi – 110025, India

103 Penang Road, #05–06/07, Visioncrest Commercial, Singapore 238467

Cambridge University Press is part of Cambridge University Press & Assessment, a department of the University of Cambridge.

We share the University's mission to contribute to society through the pursuit of education, learning and research at the highest international levels of excellence.

www.cambridge.org
Information on this title: www.cambridge.org/9781009011266

DOI: 10.1017/9781009019446

© Cambridge University Press & Assessment 2014, 2024

First published 2014
Second edition 2024

*A catalogue record for this publication is available from the British Library*

ISBN    978-1-009-01126-6    Paperback

Cambridge University Press & Assessment has no responsibility for the persistence or accuracy of URLs for external or third-party internet websites referred to in this publication and does not guarantee that any content on such websites is, or will remain, accurate or appropriate.

..............................................................................................................

Every effort has been made in preparing this book to provide accurate and up-to-date information which is in accord with accepted standards and practice at the time of publication. Although case histories are drawn from actual cases, every effort has been made to disguise the identities of the individuals involved. Nevertheless, the authors, editors and publishers can make no warranties that the information contained herein is totally free from error, not least because clinical standards are constantly changing through research and regulation. The authors, editors and publishers therefore disclaim all liability for direct or consequential damages resulting from the use of material contained in this book. Readers are strongly advised to pay careful attention to information provided by the manufacturer of any drugs or equipment that they plan to use.

# Contents

# Contributors

George Attilakos, Department of Obstetrics & Gynaecology, University College London, United Kingdom

Rachna Bahl, Department of Obstetrics & Gynaecology, St Michael's Hospital, University Hospitals Bristol NHS Foundation Trust, United Kingdom

Sadia Bhatti, Department of Obstetrics & Gynaecology, King's College Hospital London, United Kingdom

George Bugg, Department of Obstetrics & Gynaecology, Nottingham University Hospitals NHS Trust, United Kingdom

Kim Hinshaw, Department of Obstetrics and Gynaecology, City Hospitals Sunderland NHS Foundation Trust, United Kingdom

David M Levy, Department of Anaesthesia, Nottingham University Hospitals NHS Trust, United Kingdom

Shilpa Mahadasu, Department of Obstetrics and Gynaecology, South Tees Hospitals NHS Foundation Trust, United Kingdom

Glen L Mola, Department of Obstetrics and Gynaecology, School of Medicine and Health Sciences, University of Papua New Guinea, Papua New Guinea

Deirdre J Murphy, Academic Department of Obstetrics & Gynaecology, Trinity College, University of Dublin; Coombe Women & Infants University Hospital, Republic of Ireland

Patrick O'Brien, Department of Obstetrics & Gynaecology, University College Hospital London, United Kingdom

Stephen O'Brien, Department of Obstetrics & Gynaecology, Southmead Hospital, North Bristol NHS Trust, United Kingdom

Karl SJ Oláh, Department of Obstetrics & Gynaecology, South Warwickshire NHS Trust, United Kingdom

Milena Petrovic, Department of Obstetrics & Gynaecology, University College Hospital London, United Kingdom

Rowena Pykett, Department of Obstetrics & Gynaecology, Nottingham University Hospitals, United Kingdom

Meenakshi Ramphul, Department of Obstetrics & Gynaecology, Rotunda Hospital, Republic of Ireland

Dimitrios Siassakos, Department of Obstetrics & Gynaecology, University College Hospital London, United Kingdom

Bryony Strachan, Department of Obstetrics & Gynaecology, St Michael's Hospital, University Hospitals Bristol NHS Foundation Trust, United Kingdom

Derek Tuffnell, Department of Obstetrics & Gynaecology, Bradford Hospitals, United Kingdom (not practising)

Aldo Vacca, Department of Obstetrics & Gynaecology, Mater Hospital, Brisbane, Australia (not practising)

# Preface

In order to ensure we provide the highest quality of care to women, RCOG sets high standards in training. The emphasis is to ensure that the future specialists acquire both technical and non-technical skills, which together are essential to correctly manage patients within a well-functioning team of professionals. Providing training with these aims is at the forefront of RCOG educational objectives. This book provides those who are learning new skills to gain from experts' knowledge and experience. The associated course allows those in training to gain technical and non-technical skills, using simulation, in a safe environment and will ultimately improve the care offered to women.

Dr Clare McKenzie
RCOG Vice President (Education)

This book is intended for trainees attending the RCOG Assisted Birth Simulation Training (ROBuST) course. The individual chapters have been commissioned from nationally and internationally recognised experts, and adheres to and reflects current RCOG guidance around techniques in assisted vaginal birth.

Whilst we are very proud of this book, and the contents of the lectures within the course, assisted vaginal birth can only be learned with repeated, high-quality simulation sessions where the learner is at the centre of the experience and has the time and space to completely familiarise themselves with the technique. Following this, they need to be supported with facilitative hands-on teaching in real cases, allowing them to cement the practical procedure and slowly gain the confidence they need to perform the task independently.

As trainers and obstetricians we sincerely hope that you find this book and the course useful, and use it as a base from which to build your scope of practice and become one of the next generation of accoucheurs, utilising your skills to enable women and babies to have the best outcomes possible.

Dr Stephen O'Brien
Lead Editor and RCOG National Lead for Assisted Vaginal Birth Training

# Acknowledgements

The editors would like to thank the Product Development and Marketing Executive of the Royal College of Obstetricians and Gynaecologists (RCOG) who accepted the proposal for this educational text and course.

We are grateful to the individual chapter authors for sharing their expert knowledge and skills in the production of the core text and training course.

We would also like to show our gratitude to the obstetricians and gynaecologists who contributed to the development of the course and this manual, from the first iteration to this edition:

- Matthew Prior
- Rasha Mohammed
- Jennifer Browne
- Sarah Newell
- Helen van der Nelson
- Fiona Day
- Katie Cornthwaite
- Tamara Kubba
- Priya Sokhal
- Tim Draycott
- Cathy Winter

Finally, we would like to thank all the trainers who will deliver this training course on behalf of RCOG in the future.

George Attilakos, Sharon Jordan, Michelle Mojaher, Glen Mola, Stephen O'Brien and Dimitrios Siassakos

# Abbreviations

ACOG ................ American College of Obstetricians and Gynecologists

AVB .................... assisted vaginal birth

BMI .................... body mass index

BPD .................... biparietal diameter

CEFM ................ continuous electronic fetal monitoring

CPD .................... cephalopelvic disproportion

CS ...................... caesarean section

CSF .................... cerebrospinal fluid

CTG .................... cardiotocography

DDI .................... decision to delivery interval

DOA .................. direct occipito-anterior

DOP .................. direct occipito-posterior

EFM .................... electronic fetal monitoring

FBS .................... fetal blood samples

GA ...................... general anaesthesia

HIE .................... hypoxic-ischaemic encephalopathy

ICU .................... intensive care unit

ITU .................... infrapubic translabial ultrasound

LA ...................... local anaesthetic

NHSLA ................ National Health Service Litigation Authority

NICE .................. National Institute for Health and Care Excellence

OA ...................... occipito-anterior

OP ...................... occipito-posterior

OT ...................... occipito-transverse

RCOG ................ Royal College of Obstetricians and Gynaecologists

VTE .................... venous thromboembolism

WHO .................. World Health Organization

# Chapter 1
# Trends in Assisted Vaginal Birth and Future Practice

Stephen O'Brien, George Attilakos, Kim Hinshaw and Dimitrios Siassakos

## Introduction

In skilled hands, assisted vaginal birth (AVB) remains the most efficient and effective method of expediting birth in the second stage of labour. It is associated with fewer adverse maternal and neonatal outcomes compared to second stage emergency caesarean section. In this chapter we will focus on the history and role of AVB as it currently stands. We will review relevant literature, examine important areas of practice and suggest a way forward that aims to maintain AVB at the heart of obstetric practice in the twenty-first century. The need for such focus is clear – complications in the second stage of labour (fetal compromise, obstructed labour, maternal exhaustion, or maternal medical conditions exacerbated by the act of pushing) remain a major cause of maternal and neonatal mortality and morbidity across the world. Such complications are responsible for 4 to 13% of maternal deaths in Africa, Asia, Latin America and the Caribbean.[1] In 2013 obstructed labour alone accounted for 0.4 deaths per 100,000 women worldwide.[2]

### Current Practice

Since its introduction to routine clinical practice, AVB has been the preferred approach used by the accoucheur seeking to reduce maternal and neonatal morbidity in the second stage of labour.[3] In a matched cohort study, compared to assisted vaginal delivery, caesarean section (CS) at full cervical dilatation was associated with higher rates of major haemorrhage >1 L (RR 2.8; 95% CI 1.1 to 7.6) and extended hospital stay ≥6 days (RR 3.5; 95% CI 1.6 to 7.6). Neonatal

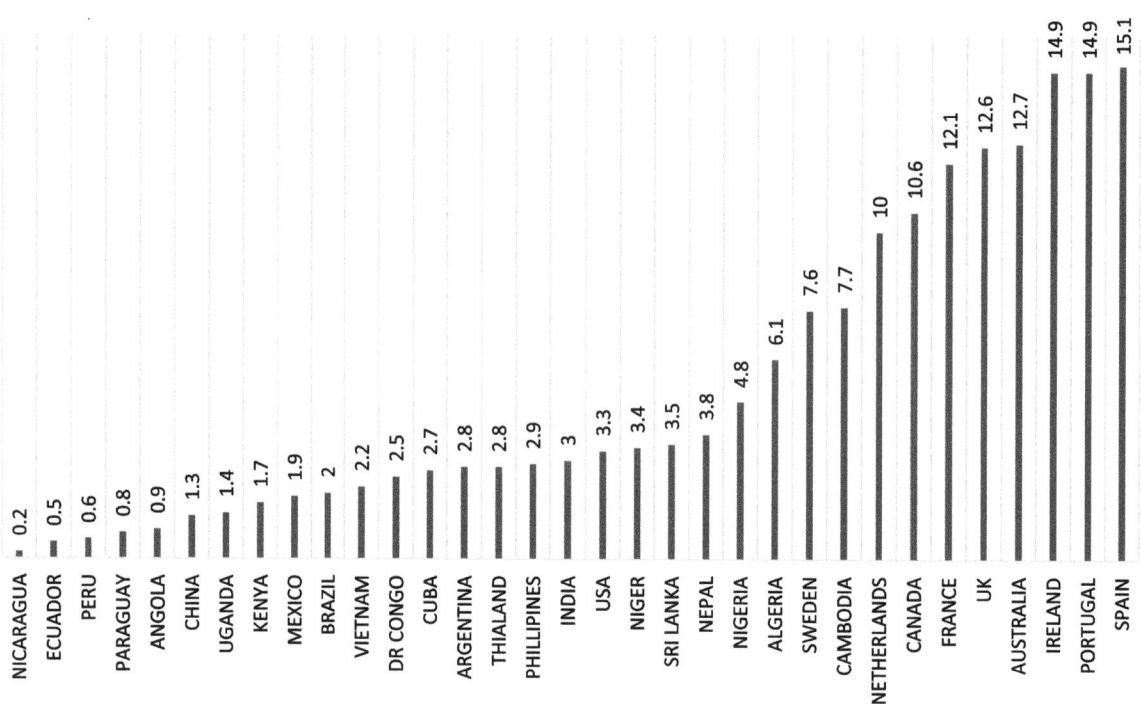

**Figure 1.1** Percentage of births as AVBs in selected countries, 2008 to 2015.

outcomes with second stage CS showed higher rates of admission for intensive care (RR 2.6; 95% CI 1.2 to 6.0) but lower rates of neonatal trauma (RR 0.4; 95% CI 0.2 to 0.7) compared to forceps.[4]

Despite this evidence suggesting an overall benefit for AVB, rates and methods of AVB have remained highly variable over time and between countries. AVB is currently performed with varying frequency in both high- and low-income countries (see Figure 1.1).[5-8]

In addition to widespread low levels of utilisation, some surveys found many areas where AVB was not used at all. In 2006 this was the case in 74% (17/23) of Latin American and Caribbean countries, 30% of countries in sub-Saharan Africa and 40% of countries in Asia.[9]

## AVB in High-Income Countries

Rates of AVB appear to have remained broadly stable within many high-income countries, although the utilisation of forceps versus ventouse/vacuum delivery has changed over time, with forceps declining and the rate of ventouse/vacuum increasing in many settings. In the UK in 1980, the overall AVB rate was 12%, with 11.3% of all births being performed with forceps but only 0.7% being performed by ventouse/vacuum.[10] By 2022 the overall rate of AVB was 11.4%, with 7% of all births performed by forceps and 4.4% performed

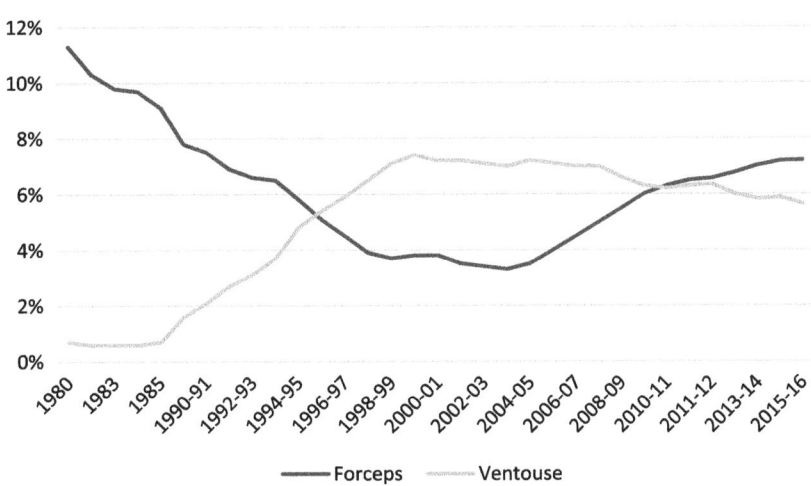

**Figure 1.2** Percentage of births performed with forceps and ventouse in the UK, 1980 to 2016.

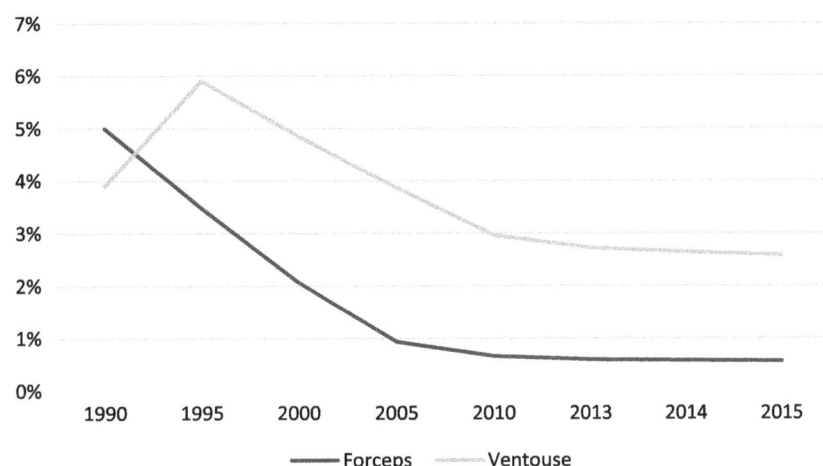

**Figure 1.3** Percentage of births performed with forceps and ventouse in the USA, 1990 to 2015.

by ventouse/vacuum.[11] This trend is shown in Figure 1.2 (data adapted from NHS Maternity Statistics, annually from 1980 to 2016).

There has been a similar change in Australia, where from 1991 to 2013 the overall AVB rate increased from 12.5% to 18%, with forceps deliveries reducing from 10% of births to 7%, while ventouse/vacuum increased from 2.5% to 11%.[5,12] In the USA, AVB rates for both forceps and ventouse/ vacuum have consistently declined in the past 30 years, from a level broadly comparable with European countries (9% of all births in 1990) to a current low of 3.12% in 2015, of which forceps were only 0.56% – see Figure 1.3 (data adapted from CDC, National Vital Statistics Reports, 2017).[13]

Since 2015, the CDC no longer makes assisted vaginal birth data routinely available, given its infrequent nature within the USA.

# Current Instruments for AVB and Associated Outcomes

Non-rotational forceps (Simpson, Rhodes, Neville-Barnes, Anderson, Wrigleys, etc.), manual rotation (usually completed with non-rotational forceps), solid mushroom cup ventouse/vacuum (Malström, Bird and Kiwi) and rotational forceps (Kielland's forceps) are the obstetric instruments currently in use. Bell cup ventouse/vacuum (silastic/silicone) are used less frequently. Other instruments (e.g. Odon) are still being developed and tested with uncertain applicability. The instruments are associated with different relative benefits and adverse outcomes. These depend not only on specific differences between devices, but also on the different clinical presentations in which the instrument is used (e.g. non-rotational versus rotational births). The different risk/benefit profile for each device, and variable experience in their use, impact on the utilisation rates of individual instruments, as well as the decision whether to attempt AVB or proceed directly to caesarean section.

## Non-rotational Instrumental Births

A non-rotational birth is an AVB where the fetal head is not rotated (or rotated <45°) by the accoucheur (either actively – i.e. rotational forceps/manual rotation, or passively – i.e. rotational ventouse/vacuum). Non-rotational births can be performed using non-rotational forceps, solid mushroom cup or bell ventouse/vacuum. Of these, forceps tend to be more successful and associated with less harm to the baby, but are potentially associated with higher maternal morbidity. The most recent Cochrane Review of 10 randomised trials involving 2,923 women showed that the use of forceps was associated with a lower risk of failure as the primary instrument (RR 0.58; CI 0.39 to 0.88) compared to ventouse/vacuum.[14] While this is an important finding given the significantly higher rates of maternal and neonatal adverse outcomes associated with the use of sequential instruments, other significant differences need to be considered; thus relative to ventouse/vacuum, forceps is:

■ Less likely to be associated with a low Apgar score at 5 minutes (<7) (RR 1.71, CI 0.59 to 4.95)

■ More likely to be associated with an umbilical arterial pH < 7.2 (RR 1.33, CI 0.91 to 1.93)

■ More likely to be associated with third/fourth degree anal sphincter injury (RR 1.83, CI 1.32 to 2.55)

■ More likely to be associated with post-partum haemorrhage (>500ml) (RR 1.7, CI 0.59 to 4.95)[14]

■ Possibly less likely to be associated with higher long-term morbidity as a result of pelvic organ prolapse, although this association has not been shown in recent population-level studies.[15,16]

Despite the apparent superiority of forceps in non-rotational birth for most maternal and neonatal outcomes, their use is generally lower worldwide than ventouse/vacuum.[17]

## Rotational Births

A rotational birth is an AVB where the fetal head is rotated by the accoucheur **by >45°** (either actively – i.e. rotational forceps/manual rotation, or passively – i.e. rotational ventouse/vacuum). Rotational births can be performed using mushroom cup ventouse/vacuum (Bird or Kiwi cup), manual rotation followed by direct forceps (or ventouse/vacuum) or rotational forceps.

Rotational births have long been perceived as being proportionately more risky than non-rotational AVBs.[18] Reflecting this, the most recent RCOG guideline specifies that rotational deliveries should be conducted in the presence of an experienced operator and in a setting with immediate recourse to caesarean section.[19] Although some small studies in previous decades have shown poorer neonatal outcomes following attempted rotational forceps births (relative to caesarean section),[20] more recent, larger studies suggest that attempted rotational birth (using any of the three approaches) is not inherently more risky than the alternative of second stage caesarean section,[21] and generates comparable outcomes to non-rotational AVB.[22,23] This has generated a renewed interest in rotational AVB for the management of malposition of the fetal head at full cervical dilatation.[24–26]

Debate continues about the most effective instrument for rotation and delivery of the fetal head. Whilst the relative efficacy of all three approaches has only been compared in one retrospective cohort study,[22] other studies have examined outcomes of various combinations of two of the three approaches.[23–25]

A large prospective randomised trial is under way in the UK (ROTATE) to examine the outcome of different rotational methods (manual, rotational forceps, rotational ventouse).

## Rotational Forceps versus Rotational Ventouse/Vacuum

In single centre trials, rotational forceps appear to be more effective compared to rotational ventouse/vacuum in terms of successful vaginal delivery. A meta-analysis in 2015 analysed eight studies (seven retrospective cohort studies and one prospective cohort study, total 2,399 patients) and reported a statistically significant reduction in the risk of failure to deliver with the intended instrument using rotational forceps compared to rotational ventouse/vacuum (RR 0.32; 95% CI 0.14 to 0.76; $p = 0.009$), with no significant differences found in any adverse maternal or neonatal outcomes.[26] However, a national audit in the UK showed the same success rate with either rotational forceps or rotational ventouse/vacuum (79%, REDEFINE, unpublished data).

## Rotational Forceps versus Manual Rotation Followed by Direct Forceps

Two UK-based retrospective cohort studies have directly compared rotational forceps with manual rotation followed by direct forceps, but they reached different conclusions: Bahl et al. found no differences in any maternal or neonatal outcomes,[22] whilst the study published by O'Brien et al. found a significantly higher chance of vaginal birth using rotational forceps than with manual rotation followed by direct forceps (RR 1.17; CI 1.04 to 1.31, p = 0.017). Additionally, birth by rotational forceps was associated with a significantly higher rate of shoulder dystocia (RR 2.35; CI 1.23 to 4.47, p = 0.012), but with no other differences in maternal or neonatal injuries.[24] Both of these studies were limited by their design (retrospective cohort) and the setting (both studies were restricted to one unit in the same city (Bristol, UK)). Moreover, the number of accoucheurs performing the rotational forceps births in each study was low (three accoucheurs in O'Brien et al.)[24] and this may limit the generalisability of the study findings.

## Manual Rotation Followed by Direct Forceps versus Rotational Ventouse/Vacuum

In 2013, in a retrospective study of 263 women, Bahl et al. compared success rates of manual rotation (followed by direct forceps) with rotational ventouse/vacuum and found no significant differences in any outcomes.[22]

Despite renewed interest, the performance of rotational AVB remains relatively specialised.

# The Way Forward for AVB

In skilled hands and in the majority of cases, AVB remains the safest and most effective means of expediting delivery in the second stage of labour. Multiple pressures, including availability of training, women's perceptions and concerns surrounding long-term complications, have acted as negative drivers on rates of AVB in many settings, across many countries. Multiple efforts by national and international bodies have not succeeded in preventing the continued rise in caesarean sections in the second stage of labour, and substantial changes to training schedules for junior obstetricians appear unlikely.

Outwith new technologies and large trials, there are approaches which can be used to promote competent and confident use of AVB. For AVB to be used regularly, both individual practitioners and healthcare units need to be confident that the techniques are being deployed safely and effectively. Women and their families need to be active participants in the decision-making, ideally through ample provision of antenatal information, well in advance of labour, as to the options to deliver a baby with malposition. Regular positive feedback, when appropriate, can be a driver that helps to both develop and maintain skills. Real time reporting and collation of outcomes can be useful. This approach, using statistical control charts of simple 'success' or 'failure' outcomes for attempted ventouse/vacuum deliveries, has been demonstrated to be a useful tool with which to target training within a large teaching unit in the UK.[27] Reporting and active review of real time outcomes has been practised routinely in surgical specialties in the UK since 2013,[28] and large population-based studies have found that this did not lead to a change in surgical patient selection or 'gaming' of the system.[29]

In a similar way, it may be useful to encourage real time open reporting of selected outcomes following attempted AVB. Trainees would benefit from confirmation of developing or continued competence, allowing them to grow in confidence and become more assured of their skills. Trainers and hosting hospitals would be able to use the data generated to pick up early when individuals are not meeting expected thresholds of competence. This would allow for focused, targeted training, and correction of 'less than ideal' practices at an early stage.

Feedback from women and their families is also necessary and will increase both the perceived and the actual safety of AVB.

AVB has long been considered to be the essential core skill that every obstetrician should be able to confidently offer. Developing and maintaining relevant skills in AVB should continue, supported by an ongoing research base and continuous audit of practice. This will ensure safe, effective and appropriate use of all available AVB techniques.

# References

1.  Khan KS, Wojdyla D, Say L, Gülmezoglu AM, Look PFV. WHO analysis of causes of maternal death: a systematic review. The Lancet. 2006;367(9516):1066–74.

2.  GBD 2013 Mortality and Causes of Death Collaborators. Global, regional, and national age-sex specific all-cause and cause-specific mortality for 240 causes of death, 1990–2013: a systematic analysis for the Global Burden of Disease Study 2013. The Lancet. 2015;385(9963):117–71.

3.  Arulkumaran S, Robson M. *Munro Kerr's Operative Obstetrics*. 13th ed. Arulkumaran S, Robson M, editors. London: Elsevier; 2019.

4.  Murphy DJ, Liebling RE, Verity L, Swingler R, Patel R. Early maternal and neonatal morbidity associated with operative delivery in second stage of labour: a cohort study. The Lancet. 2001; 358(9289):1203–7.

5.  AIHW. Australian mothers and babies 2015 – in brief. 2017; p. 1–72.

6.  Macfarlane AJ, Blondel B, Mohangoo AD et al. Wide differences in mode of delivery within Europe: risk-stratified analyses of aggregated routine data from the Euro-Peristat study. BJOG: An International Journal of Obstetrics & Gynaecology. 2016;123(4):559–68.

7.  National Centre for Health Statistics. Births: Final Data for 2013. 2015;64(1):1–68.

8.  Souza JP, Gülmezoglu A, Lumbiganon P et al. caesarean section without medical indications is associated with an increased risk of adverse short-term maternal outcomes: the 2004–2008 WHO Global Survey on Maternal and Perinatal Health. BMC Medicine. 2010;8:71.

9.  Fauveau V. Is vacuum extraction still known, taught and practiced? A worldwide KAP survey. International Journal of Gynecology and Obstetrics. 2006;94(2):185–9.

10. General Statistical Service, NHS Maternity Statistics, England: 1980–1994. 1998; p. 1–43.

11. NHS Digital. NHS Maternity Statistics, England – 2021–22 [Internet]. London: NHS Digital; 2022 [accessed 15 March 2023]. https://digital.nhs.uk/data-and-information/publications/statistical/nhs-maternity-statistics/2021-22

12. AIHW. Australia's Mothers and Babies 1991. 1994; p. 1–84.

13. CDC. National Vital Statistics Reports, Volume 66, Number 1, January 5, 2017. Dec p. 1–70.

14. Verma GL, Spalding JJ, Wilkinson MD et al. Instruments for assisted vaginal birth. Cochrane Db Syst Rev. 2021;2021(9):CD005455.

15. Barber M. Pervasive impacts of mode of delivery across multiple measures of prolapse severity. BJOG: An International Journal of Obstetrics & Gynaecology. 2015;123(9):1557.

16. Volløyhaug I, Mørkved S, Salvesen Ø, Salvesen K. Pelvic organ prolapse and incontinence 15–23 years after first delivery: a cross-sectional study. BJOG: An International Journal of Obstetrics & Gynaecology. 2015;122(7):964–71.

17. Deering S. Forceps, simulation, and social media. Obstetrics & Gynecology. 2016 Sep;128(3):425–6.

18. Patel RR. Forceps delivery in modern obstetric practice. BMJ (Clinical research ed.). 2004;328(7451):1302–5.

19. Murphy DJ, Strachan BK, Bahl R. . Assisted Vaginal Birth: Green-top Guideline No. 26. BJOG: An International Journal of Obstetrics & Gynaecology. 2020.

20. Chiswick ML, James DK. Kielland's forceps: association with neonatal morbidity and mortality. BMJ (Clinical research ed.). 1979;1(6155):7–9.

21. Aiken AR, Aiken CE, Alberry MS, Brockelsby JC, Scott JG. Management of fetal malposition in the second stage of labor: a propensity score analysis. American Journal of Obstetrics and Gynecology [Internet]. 2015 ;212(3):355.e1-355.e7.

22. Bahl R, Venne MV de, Macleod M, Strachan B, Murphy DJ. Maternal and neonatal morbidity in relation to the instrument used for mid-cavity rotational operative vaginal delivery: a prospective

cohort study. BJOG: An International Journal of Obstetrics & Gynaecology. 2013 Aug 7;120(12):1526–33.

23. Tempest N, Hart A, Walkinshaw S, Hapangama DK. A re-evaluation of the role of rotational forceps: retrospective comparison of maternal and perinatal outcomes following different methods of birth for malposition in the second stage of labour. BJOG: An International Journal of Obstetrics & Gynaecology [Internet]. 2013;120(10):1277–84.

24. O'Brien S, Day F, Lenguerrand E et al. Rotational forceps versus manual rotation and direct forceps: a retrospective cohort study. European Journal of Obstetrics, Gynecology, and Reproductive Biology. 2017;212:119–25.

25. Al-Suhel R, Gill S, Robson S, Shadbolt B. Kielland's forceps in the new millennium. Maternal and neonatal outcomes of attempted rotational forceps delivery. Australian and New Zealand Journal of Obstetrics and Gynaecology. 2009 ;49(5):510–4.

26. Wattar BHA, Wattar BA, Gallos I, Pirie AM. Rotational vaginal delivery with Kielland's forceps. Current Opinion in Obstetrics and Gynaecology. 2015;27(6):438–44.

27. Lane S, Weeks A, Scholefield H. Monitoring obstetricians' performance with statistical process control charts. BJOG: An International Journal of Obstetrics & Gynaecology. 2007;114(5):614–8.

28. NHS England. Everyone Counts: Planning for Patients 2013/14 [Internet]. 2012

29. Vallance AE, Fearnhead NS, Kuryba A et al. Effect of public reporting of surgeons' outcomes on patient selection, 'gaming,' and mortality in colorectal cancer surgery in England: population based cohort study. BMJ (Clinical research ed.). 2018;361:k1581.

# Chapter 2
# Indications and Assessment for Assisted Vaginal Birth

Deirdre Murphy and Meenakshi Ramphul

## Introduction

The decision whether or not to recommend an assisted vaginal birth (AVB) is a complex one. Decision-making about the most appropriate mode of birth needs to take account of the key elements for a safe AVB which are that it needs to be conducted under optimal circumstances, in the most appropriate place and by a competent operator. Safety issues need to be balanced with the aim of providing a positive birth experience for the mother and her partner. The risks of maternal and neonatal morbidity are increased with AVBs, although with appropriate case selection and careful practice these risks are low.[1] Careful attention needs to be paid to the indication for AVB and to clinical assessment prior to any attempt at a procedure.

There are two alternatives to AVB. The first, continued pushing aiming for a spontaneous vaginal birth, may be preferred by women when progress is being made and the fetal status is satisfactory. However, an expectant approach may be unwise if there is evidence of fetal compromise (meconium, abnormal fetal heart rate, low pH) or diminished maternal reserve (exhaustion and absence of progress). The second approach, a caesarean section at full dilatation, is a complex surgical procedure associated with increased risks of maternal morbidity (major haemorrhage, extended hospital stay) and neonatal morbidity (higher rates of admission to the neonatal unit).[2] Overall, women who have vaginal births (even with assistance) tend to be more satisfied with the birth than those who have emergency caesarean sections. The risk of intrapartum complications in subsequent pregnancies is greatly reduced if a vacuum or forceps-assisted delivery can be completed safely.[3,4]

# Classification of Assisted Vaginal Birth

Vacuum and forceps-assisted deliveries are classified primarily by the station and position of the fetal head (see Table 2.1). The station of the fetal head refers to descent of the leading part of the skull within the birth canal in relation to the maternal ischial spines.[5] The position refers to the orientation of the fetal occiput (the denominator in a vertex presentation) in relation to the maternal pubic symphysis. The fetal station must be at the level of the ischial spines (station 0) or below to fulfil the criteria for safe AVB. In most circumstances, this correlates with none of the fetal head palpable abdominally (zero fifths, a deeply engaged presenting part). The exception is with a deflexed occipito-posterior (OP) position of the fetal head at the level of the ischial spines (station 0), where there may be up to (but no more than) one-fifth of the fetal head palpable abdominally for AVB to be considered mid-pelvic and therefore potentially suitable for vacuum or forceps-assisted delivery. Occipito-anterior (OA) positions are less challenging for AVB than occipito-transverse (OT) or OP positions (fetal malpositions). Assisted vaginal births are therefore subclassified into those that require or those that do not require rotation.

A standard classification should be used to enable clear communication, benchmarking, audit and comparisons between studies. The Royal College of Obstetricians and Gynaecologists (RCOG) uses adapted criteria from the guidelines of the American College of Obstetricians and Gynecologists (ACOG) (see Table 2.1).[6,7] The first important stage in training obstetricians for AVB is

**Table 2.1** Classification for assisted vaginal birth

| | |
|---|---|
| **Outlet** | Fetal scalp visible without separating the labia<br>Fetal skull has reached the perineum<br>Rotation does not exceed 45° |
| **Low** | Fetal skull is at station +2 cm, but not on the perineum<br>Two subdivisions:<br>1. non-rotational ≤ 45°<br>2. rotational > 45° |
| **Mid** | Fetal head is no more than one-fifth palpable per abdomen<br>Leading point of the skull is at station 0 or +1 cm<br>Two subdivisions:<br>1. non-rotational ≤ 45°<br>2. rotational > 45° |

to ensure consistency and accuracy in assessment of the station and position of the fetal head, and therefore in classification of the planned procedure. The supervising obstetrician should be confident that this competency has been achieved before indirect supervision is provided.

# Indications

Assisted vaginal births are performed when delivery needs to be expedited and may be indicated by the condition of the fetus or the mother or both. The overall premise should be to recommend AVB when the benefits are thought to outweigh the risks.

The most common indication for AVB is slow progress in the second stage of labour. In nulliparous women, a delay in the second stage with regional anaesthesia is diagnosed when delivery is not imminent after three hours from the diagnosis of full cervical dilatation (total passive and active second stage) or after two hours without regional anaesthesia. In multiparous women, this delay is diagnosed when delivery is not imminent after two hours with regional anaesthesia (total passive and active second stage) or one hour without regional anaesthesia.[8] The basis for these time limits is largely empirical rather than evidence-based; therefore clinical judgement is required when applying time limits. It should be recognised that where a woman has been pushing effectively for 30 (parous) to 60 minutes (nulliparous) with no discernible progress, earlier assessment (but not necessarily intervention) may be appropriate as a fetal malposition (OT/OP), malpresentation (brow/face) or cephalopelvic disproportion (CPD) may be present. In these circumstances, an assessment should be sought from a senior clinician with regard to ongoing management, rather than persisting for two hours or more with unproductive pushing that may exacerbate the problem.

Suspected fetal compromise, as suggested by a non-reassuring or pathological fetal heart rate pattern on cardiotocography (CTG), meconium or a low pH on fetal blood sampling (FBS), is also a common indication for AVB. Special fetal circumstances include suspected sepsis (maternal pyrexia, maternal tachycardia, fetal tachycardia, foul-smelling amniotic fluid), intrauterine growth restriction, preterm labour, intrapartum vaginal bleeding, labour following a previous caesarean section, and fetal heart rate abnormalities in a second twin. In these circumstances, the fetal reserve may be diminished and the decision to intervene should take account of the potential for a more rapidly developing hypoxia in the fetus.

Maternal indications for AVB include medical conditions that preclude prolonged maternal effort such as maternal cardiac disease, hypertensive crisis, cerebrovascular disease or respiratory compromise.

Most indications are relative and there may be more than one indication to perform an AVB, for example, prolonged pushing in the second stage of labour is frequently complicated by CTG abnormalities. When to intervene is therefore a balance of risks and benefits and will depend on individual clinical circumstances and maternal preferences.

## Contra-indications

Assisted vaginal births are contra-indicated when the cervix is less than ten centimetres dilated and when the fetal head is not fully engaged (station above the ischial spines and/or more than one-fifth of the fetal head palpable abdominally) (see Table 2.2). AVBs are relatively contra-indicated in cases of fetal bleeding disorders (e.g. suspected thrombocytopenia) or a predisposition to fracture (e.g. osteogenesis imperfecta). However, in some circumstances, it may be more traumatic for the fetus to be delivered abdominally than vaginally, for example, in advanced labour with the fetal head deep in the pelvis. In cases of blood-borne viral infections such as Hepatitis B/C and HIV, AVBs are not contra-indicated, but as there is an increased risk of fetal abrasion or scalp trauma, it is sensible to avoid potentially difficult mid-pelvic or rotational procedures.

Forceps can be used for some malpresentations such as face presentation in the mento-anterior position or for the after-coming head of the breech where maternal effort is impossible or contra-indicated. In cases of brow or a mento-posterior face presentation, AVB should not be attempted unless the brow can be flexed to a vertex presentation or deflexed to a face presentation, and the mento-posterior face presentation requires rotation to mento-anterior. These procedures require specialist expertise and are not suitable for novice practitioners.

Vacuum deliveries are contra-indicated for preterm deliveries at gestations of less than 32 completed weeks due to the increased risk of cephalohaematoma, intracranial haemorrhage, subgaleal haemorrhage and neonatal jaundice. It has also been suggested that the vacuum extractor should be avoided at less than 36 completed weeks gestation; however this is controversial with limited data to establish the safety of the vacuum extractor at gestations between 32 and 36 weeks. As

**Table 2.2** Safety criteria for assisted vaginal birth

| | |
|---|---|
| Full abdominal and vaginal examination | ■ Head is ≤1/5 palpable per abdomen (in most cases not palpable)<br>■ Cervix is fully dilated and the membranes are ruptured<br>■ Station at level of ischial spines or below<br>■ Position of the fetal head has been determined<br>■ Caput and moulding are no more than moderate (or +2)[a]<br>■ Pelvis is deemed adequate |
| Preparation of mother | ■ Clear explanation given, and informed consent taken and documented in woman's case notes<br>■ Trust established and full cooperation sought and agreed with woman<br>■ Appropriate analgesia is in place: for mid-pelvic or rotational birth, this will usually be a regional block; a pudendal block may be acceptable depending on urgency; and a perineal block may be sufficient for low or outlet birth<br>■ Aseptic technique<br>■ Maternal bladder has been emptied<br>■ Indwelling catheter has been removed or balloon deflated |
| Preparation of staff | ■ Operator has the knowledge, experience and skill necessary<br>■ Adequate facilities are available (equipment, bed, lighting) and access to an operating theatre<br>■ Backup plan: for mid-pelvic births, theatre facilities should be available to allow a caesarean birth to be performed without delay; a senior obstetrician should be present if an inexperienced obstetrician is conducting the birth<br>■ Anticipation of complications that may arise (e.g. shoulder dystocia, perineal trauma, postpartum haemorrhage)<br>■ Personnel present who are trained in neonatal resuscitation |

[a] *Moderate moulding or +2 moulding is where the parietal bones are overlapped but easily reduced; severe moulding or +3 is where the parietal bones have overlapped and are irreducible indicating cephalopelvic disproportion.*

a general rule, most obstetricians avoid vacuum delivery at gestations less than 36 completed weeks.

Maternal consent is a prerequisite for AVB; therefore refusing consent to vacuum or forceps-assisted delivery is a contra-indication. The alternatives and associated risks must be clearly outlined to the woman and her partner. Prolonged pushing may be detrimental to the fetus, particularly in cases of suspected fetal compromise or uncertain fetal reserve. Similarly, the woman needs to be aware that there is increased maternal and neonatal morbidity associated with caesarean section at full dilatation when performed with the head deep in the pelvis, and this may be more traumatic than an AVB.[2] Ideally these discussions should take place in the antenatal period or earlier in the course of the labour if limitations have been expressed or documented in a birth plan. A similar approach is required where a woman has stated a preference for a particular choice of instrument.

# Prerequisites

Before performing an AVB, a careful assessment of the clinical situation, clear communication with the mother, partner and healthcare personnel, and expertise in the planned procedure are essential (see Table 2.2).

The indication for the procedure should be established and clearly documented. Informed consent should be obtained from the woman after explicit counselling regarding the indication, advantages and disadvantages and nature of the procedure. This may be difficult to achieve in what is essentially an emergency setting, but information should be given to the woman between contractions and the birth plan of the mother should be taken into account and discussed. The principles of obtaining valid consent in labour should be followed and consent advice from the RCOG on AVBs should be followed.[6]

The alternatives to an AVB – continued pushing or caesarean section – should also be discussed with the woman, outlining the advantages and disadvantages of each option. For AVBs in the delivery room, verbal consent should be obtained and clearly documented in the notes, with an endeavour to obtain written consent when possible. However, for AVBs in theatre (conducted as a 'trial'), written consent should be obtained.[6]

A systematic abdominal and vaginal examination should be performed to establish an estimate of the size of the fetus, the engagement, position, station and attitude of the fetal head, the pelvic dimensions and the adequacy of analgesia, as outlined in Assessment Prior to Assisted Vaginal Birth below. For low or outlet deliveries, infiltration of local anaesthetic into the perineum may suffice but a pudendal block may be required, particularly for forceps. For mid-pelvic deliveries, especially rotational procedures, regional anaesthesia (epidural or spinal) is optimal. Prior to the procedure, the bladder should be emptied by 'in and out' catheterisation to reduce the risk of urethral or bladder damage. If an indwelling catheter is already in place, the bulb should be deflated.

The operator should have the appropriate knowledge, skills and experience required. Trainees should be adequately supervised by more senior obstetricians, especially in cases of mid-pelvic or rotational deliveries. AVBs can be associated with maternal and fetal morbidity, particularly in cases of sequential use of instruments (vacuum followed by forceps) and failed AVBs (vacuum and/or forceps followed by caesarean section), which are often related to inexperience of the operator.[2,9]

# Assessment Prior to Assisted Vaginal Birth

## General Considerations

An open and positive first impression is important in building rapport and trust with the woman and her carers. The obstetrician should attempt to gauge the atmosphere and morale within the room and respond sensitively and with empathy to the woman's situation. Birth partners will sometimes advocate on behalf of the woman, but care should be taken, especially if there are communication difficulties. Professionally trained interpreters should be used wherever possible for women whose first language is not English or who are hearing impaired.

## Clinical History To Date

Before attempting an AVB, it is important to review the woman's medical and obstetric history to exclude any contra-indications to AVB and to anticipate any potential complications (e.g. CPD, shoulder dystocia, neonatal injury or postpartum haemorrhage). The past obstetric history, presence of diabetes, antenatal diagnosis of fetal concerns (abnormal growth, oligohydramnios, abnormal fetal Doppler studies, fetal anomaly) and maternal blood results (serology, anaemia, rhesus) may be of particular relevance. The partogram should be assessed, looking at progress in the first stage of labour, the efficiency of uterine contractions and the use of oxytocin. The maternal body mass index, vital signs and hydration status should be noted. Particular attention should be paid to maternal pyrexia or tachycardia.

## Review of the Fetal Status

The fetal status should be assessed as a matter of priority as this will determine the need for urgency in terms of intervention. Women identified as high-risk antenatally or in labour should be recommended continuous electronic fetal monitoring (EFM) with CTG. The four features of the fetal heart recording (baseline fetal heart rate, variability, accelerations, decelerations) and the uterine contractions (care should be taken to record uterine activity adequately) should be noted to classify the trace as normal, suspicious or pathological.[8] Any FBS taken in the first or second stage of labour should also be noted. Meconium-stained liquor should be considered as a possible sign of fetal compromise although this may be a normal finding in pregnancies that have progressed beyond term. Absence of liquor should also be considered abnormal as it may reflect undetected placental insufficiency. A degree of urgency is required for CTGs that are classified as pathological and for FBS with a pH below 7.20, particularly in the context of meconium.[8]

## Abdominal Examination

A systematic abdominal examination using Leopold's four manoeuvres should be undertaken. The fetal lie and presentation should be confirmed, and the fetal size should be assessed clinically. A small-for-gestational-age fetus is an important finding in terms of reduced fetal reserve in labour but also for ease of delivery. A clinically large-for-gestational-age fetus may be associated with CPD and a failed attempt at AVB or with shoulder dystocia and subsequent postpartum haemorrhage. Engagement of the fetal head occurs when the widest transverse diameter of the fetal head (biparietal diameter – BPD) passes through the pelvic inlet.[5] Engagement of the fetal head should be ascertained abdominally and is described in terms of 'fifths' palpable, depending on how much of the head is palpable abdominally. AVBs should only be attempted where no more than one-fifth of the head is palpable abdominally, and in the majority of cases there will be zero fifths palpable abdominally. The position of the fetal back can also be helpful to define the position of the fetal head, although in practice this is often difficult.

## Vaginal Examination

A systematic vaginal examination should be performed to confirm full cervical dilatation, a cephalic vertex presentation, the position, station and attitude (degree of flexion) of the fetal head, the degree of caput (scalp swelling) and moulding (closure and overlap of the skull bones), and to form a subjective impression of the pelvic dimensions. In addition, it is extremely helpful to assess whether rotation (if required) and descent occur during the contraction with active pushing. This is a dynamic form of assessment and is very useful in decision-making.

Palpation of each fontanelle (anterior and posterior) and the suture lines of the fetal skull should be carried out to determine the fetal head position as accurately as possible (see Figures 2.1 and 2.2). However, digital vaginal examination is not always accurate, especially in the presence of caput, moulding and asynclitism.[10,11] The accuracy of digital vaginal examination to determine the fetal head position in the second stage of labour has been compared to transabdominal ultrasound and reported to be between 35% and 80%.[10–18]

The station of the fetal head should be ascertained routinely on vaginal examination. However, similar to inaccuracy of the fetal head position, there is evidence that vaginal assessment of the station of the fetal head is not always reliable.[19] A tool investigated to improve the accuracy of assessment of the station of the fetal head is the 'StationMaster' (a modified amniotomy hook which relocates the reference point for defining the station from the ischial spines to the posterior fourchette).[20] A simulation study of the 'StationMaster' using a mannequin pelvis showed that it was more accurate than digital assessment of fetal head station.[20]

The position and station of the fetal head will be important indicators of the level of skill required of the operator and will also have an impact on the choice of instrument and where the delivery is carried out (delivery room versus operating theatre). Rotation and descent of the presenting part with uterine activity and maternal effort is a good prognostic factor for successful AVB but cases with minimal or no descent should be treated with caution. Similarly, the presence of marked caput or moulding of the fetal skull bones should be established, as irreducible moulding may be a warning sign for CPD.

## Ultrasound Assessment

Clinicians should be aware that ultrasound assessment of the fetal head position prior to AVB may be more reliable than clinical examination.[21] A multicentre RCT compared ultrasound assessment of the fetal head position prior to AVB with standard care to determine whether the use of ultrasound can reduce the incidence of incorrect diagnosis of the fetal head position. The incidence of incorrect diagnosis was significantly lower in the ultrasound group than the standard care group (4/257 [1.6%] versus 52/257 [20.2%]; OR 0.06, 95% CI 0.02–0.19; $P < 0.001$).[21] While correct diagnosis of the fetal head position is a prerequisite for a safe operative vaginal birth, the ultrasound assessment in itself did not lead to a reduction in morbidity.

A further trial evaluated ultrasound assessment of the fetal head position from 8 cm cervical dilatation compared with standard vaginal examination and reported a higher incidence of caesarean birth in the ultrasound group (7.8% versus 4.9%; RR 1.60, 95% CI 1.12–2.28), but no significant difference in rates of AVB (25.8% versus 22.2%; RR 1.16, 95% CI 0.99–1.37).[22]

A number of observational studies have reported the use of abdominal or perineal ultrasound to assess the fetal station, flexion of the head and direction of head descent in the second stage of labour.[23–25] Currently, there is insufficient standardisation of these techniques or evidence of benefit to recommend their routine use in clinical practice.

## Observation Period

Observation of the maternal effort and the woman's psychological status during active pushing often helps the operator decide when to recommend intervention and what instrument to use. The perspective of the woman and the midwife caring for her will assist the decision-making process. This may be more limited in time-sensitive emergency cases such as fetal bradycardia.

# Choice of Instruments

The choice of forceps or vacuum extractor will depend on the clinical circumstances and on the operator's competencies and preferences. Forceps-assisted delivery may be more effective in instances where there is diminished maternal effort (e.g. maternal exhaustion, dense epidural block, general anaesthesia), for preterm deliveries (<34–36 weeks gestation), after a failed attempt at vacuum extraction, for delivery of the after-coming head in breech deliveries and for low-pelvic deliveries with suspected fetal coagulopathy or thrombocytopenia. A vacuum-assisted delivery may be preferred where analgesia is limited, for low-pelvic or outlet deliveries. The relative merits of vacuum extraction and forceps have been explored in a Cochrane systematic review of RCTs[9] and are summarised in Table 2.2. The ROTATE multicentre RCT will provide evidence on the effectiveness and safety profiles of rotational methods (manual, Kielland's, vacuum) for malpositions.

## Forceps

There are at least 700 different types of forceps and there have been no RCTs comparing forceps types. The three main types (outlet, mid-pelvic and rotational) can be used in specific situations but require differing levels of expertise. Forceps are more likely than vacuum to be successful at achieving vaginal birth with a single instrument.[26] Use of a single reliable instrument will be preferable in critical cases of fetal bradycardia, cord prolapse or placental abruption.[27] However, compared to vacuum, forceps are associated with a higher incidence of pelvic floor trauma, third- or fourth-degree tears, facial injuries to the neonate and increased analgesia requirements.[28] Rotational delivery with Kielland's forceps requires specific expertise and training. Manual rotation followed by direct traction forceps may be useful, depending on the operator's skills and experience.[6]

## Vacuum

Vacuum cups can be metal, plastic or silicone. The vacuum extractor is used increasingly as the instrument of first choice. This reflects the need for less analgesia/anaesthesia and the lower incidence of maternal pelvic floor trauma.[28] However, compared to forceps delivery, vacuum extraction is associated with an increased risk of neonatal cephalhaematoma, retinal haemorrhage and maternal concern about the well-being of the neonate.[28] A Cochrane systematic review showed that the metal cup was more likely than a soft cup to result in a successful vaginal birth with no difference in maternal perineal trauma.[28] However, the metal cup was associated with an increased risk of neonatal bruising, cephalhaematoma and scalp injury. Two randomised controlled trials comparing a disposable vacuum device (Kiwi Omnicup) with standard vacuum cups reported high rates of instrument failure requiring sequential use of forceps (20 to 30%) with a significantly higher incidence with the disposable device.[29,30]

# Attempted AVB in Theatre

AVBs that are anticipated to have a higher rate of failure should be carried out in a place where immediate recourse to caesarean section can be undertaken.[6] Fetal hypoxic ischaemic injuries can occur when there is a delay between a failed attempt at AVB (especially in a delivery room) and a caesarean section. Failure rates are higher for mid-pelvic deliveries, women with a high maternal body mass index (BMI > 30 kg/m$^2$), babies with a birth weight over 4.0 kg and fetal malpositions, in particular the OP position.

Transfer to theatre for an attempted AVB with preparations in case of a caesarean section has the advantages of facilitating optimal anaesthesia, enhanced clinical assessment and, where hospital protocols are in place, senior support for the delivery. There will be a delay in the decision to delivery interval associated with transferring a woman to theatre compared to delivering in the labour room, but this has not been found to be associated with adverse neonatal outcomes.[31] The decision to transfer the woman to theatre should balance the benefits in terms of safety should AVB fail with the potential negatives in terms of delay in the decision to delivery interval, and the additional anxiety for the woman and her partner.

# Complications

Complications are an inherent risk with any surgical procedure. Appropriate use of vacuum extractors and forceps by well-trained obstetricians should minimise the risk of complications and alleviate the risks to the mother and baby of delaying delivery. However, failure to assess the clinical scenario correctly could result in avoidable maternal and neonatal morbidity. Failure to diagnose a fetal malposition increases the likelihood of failed AVB with the additional morbidity of sequential use of instruments or second stage caesarean section. Misjudging the fetal size or signs of CPD may lead to shoulder dystocia, failed AVB or fetal head impaction at caesarean section. When assessing fetal well-being, signs of sepsis or significant CTG abnormalities may be mis-interpreted resulting in neonatal hypoxic ischaemic encephalopathy (HIE) and subsequent cerebral palsy.[1,2,9]

Poorly conducted AVBs increase the likelihood of third- and fourth-degree tears, vaginal wall and cervical lacerations, postpartum haemorrhage, long term pelvic floor sequelae (prolapse and incontinence) and psychological distress. For the neonate, poorly conducted AVBs are associated with traumatic injuries, HIE, cerebral haemorrhage and rarely perinatal death. caesarean section in the second stage of labour after a failed attempt at AVB can be extremely challenging with impaction of the fetal head, extension of the uterine incision and massive obstetric haemorrhage. Operators need to be aware of the potential complications, mitigate against them and have the expertise to deal with them if they occur; and they must call for senior assistance early.

# Conclusion

AVB has an important role to play in modern obstetric care. Women who have a vacuum or forceps-assisted delivery are far more likely to have a spontaneous vaginal birth in a subsequent pregnancy than women who have an emergency caesarean section. Careful patient assessment, observing the rules of safe obstetric practice and working within the appropriate clinical indications for AVBs should ensure that the benefits of recommending AVB outweigh the risks.

# References

1.  Demissie K, Rhoads GG, Smulian JC et al. Operative vaginal delivery and neonatal and infant adverse outcomes: population based retrospective analysis. BMJ. 2004;329(7456):24–9.

2.  Murphy D, Liebling R, Verity L, Swingler R, Patel R. Cohort study of the early maternal and neonatal morbidity associated with operative delivery in the second stage of labour. Lancet. 2001 (358):1203–7.

3.  Bahl R, Strachan B, Murphy DJ. Outcome of subsequent pregnancy three years after previous operative delivery in the second stage of labour: cohort study. BMJ. 2004;328(7435):311.

4.  DiMatteo MR, Morton SC, Lepper HS et al. Cesarean childbirth and psychosocial outcomes: a meta-analysis. Health Psychol. 1996;15(4):303–14.

5.  Cunningham F, Leveno K, Bloom S et al. *Williams Obstetrics*. 23rd ed. New York: McGraw Hill, 2009.

6.  Murphy DJ, Strachan BK, Bahl R on behalf of the Royal College of Obstetricians and Gynaecologists. Assisted Vaginal Birth. BJOG. 2020; https://doi.org/10.1111/1471-0528.16092

7.  American College of Obstetricians and Gynecologists. *Practice Bulletin 17. Operative Vaginal Delivery*. Washington DC: ACOG, 2000.

8.  National Institute for Health and Clinical Excellence. *Intrapartum Care*. Clinical guideline 55. London: National Institute for Health and Clinical Excellence. 2007.

9.  Murphy D, Liebling R, Patel R, Verity L, Swingler R. Cohort study of operative delivery in the second stage of labour and standard of obstetric care. Br J Obstet Gynaecol. 2003; (110):610–5.

10. Akmal S, Tsoi E, Kametas N, Howard R, Nicolaides KH. Intrapartum sonography to determine fetal head position. J Matern Fetal Neonatal Med. 2002;12(3):172–7.

11. Dupuis O, Ruimark S, Corinne D et al. Fetal head position during the second stage of labor: comparison of digital vaginal examination and transabdominal ultrasonographic examination. Eur J Obstet Gynecol Reprod Biol. 2005;123(2):193–7.

12. Souka AP, Haritos T, Basayiannis K, Noikokyri N, Antsaklis A. Intrapartum ultrasound for the examination of the fetal head position in normal and obstructed labor. J Matern Fetal Neonatal Med. 2003;13(1):59–63.

13. Sherer DM, Miodovnik M, Bradley KS, Langer O. Intrapartum fetal head position II: comparison between transvaginal digital examination and transabdominal ultrasound assessment during the second stage of labor. Ultrasound Obstet Gynecol. 2002;19(3):264–8.

14. Kreiser D, Schiff E, Lipitz S et al. Determination of fetal occiput position by ultrasound during the second stage of labor. J Matern Fetal Neonatal Med. 2001 August;10(4):283–6.

15. Zahalka N, Sadan O, Malinger G et al. Comparison of transvaginal sonography with digital examination and transabdominal sonography for the determination of fetal head position in the second stage of labor. Am J Obstet Gynecol. 2005;193(2):381–6.

16. Chou R, Kreiser D, Taslimi M, Druzin M, El-Sayed Y. Vaginal versus ultrasound examination of fetal occiput position during the second stage of labor. Am J Obstet Gynecol. 2004;191:521–4.

17. Rozenberg P, Porcher R, Salomon LJ et al. Comparison of the learning curves of digital examination and transabdominal sonography for the determination of fetal head position during labor. Ultrasound Obstet Gynecol. 2008;31(3):332–7.

18. Ramphul M, Murphy DJ. Establishing the accuracy and acceptability of abdominal ultrasound to define the fetal head position in the second stage of labour: a validation study. Eur J Obstet Gynecol Reprod Biol. 2012.

19. Dupuis O, Silveira R, Zentner A et al. Birth simulator: reliability of transvaginal assessment of fetal head station as defined by the American College of Obstetricians and Gynecologists classification. AJOG. 2005;192(3):868–74.

20. Awan N, Rhoades A, Weeks AD. The validity and reliability of the StationMaster: a device to improve the accuracy of station assessment in labour. Eur J Obstet Gynecol Reprod Biol. 2009;145(1):65–70.

21. Ramphul M, Ooi PV, Burke G et al. Instrumental delivery and ultrasound: a multicentre randomised controlled trial of ultrasound assessment of the fetal head position versus standard care as an approach to prevent morbidity at instrumental delivery. BJOG 2014;121:1029–38.

22. Popowski T, Porcher R, Fort J, Javoise S, Rozenberg P. Influence of ultrasound determination of fetal head position on mode of delivery: a pragmatic randomized trial. Ultrasound Obstet Gynecol. 2015;46:520–5.

23. Sananes NP, Kasbaoui S, Severac F et al. 96: ultrasound measurement of the perineum-fetal head distance as a predictive factor of difficult vaginal operative delivery. Am J Obstet Gynecol. 2017;216:S69.

24. Kasbaoui S, Séverac F, Aïssi G et al. Predicting the difficulty of operative vaginal delivery by ultrasound measurement of fetal head station. Am J Obstet Gynecol. 2017;216:507.

25. Bultez T, Quibel T, Bouhanna P et al. Angle of fetal head progression measured using transperineal ultrasound as a predictive factor of vacuum extraction failure. Ultrasound Obstet Gynecol. 2016; 48:86–91.

26. Murphy D, Macleod M, Bahl R, Strachan B. A cohort study of maternal and neonatal morbidity in relation to use of sequential instruments at operative vaginal delivery. Eur J Obstet Gynecol Reprod Biol. 2011;156(1):41–5.

27. Okunwobi-Smith Y, Cooke I, MacKenzie IZ. Decision to delivery intervals for assisted vaginal vertex delivery. BJOG. 2000;107(4):467–71.

28. O'Mahony F, Hofmeyr GJ, Menon V. Choice of instruments for assisted vaginal delivery. Cochrane Database Syst Rev. 2010(11):CD005455.

29. Attilakos G, Sibanda T, Winter C, Johnson N, Draycott T. A randomised controlled trial of a new handheld vacuum extraction device. BJOG 2005;112(11):1510–5.

30. Groom KM, Jones BA, Miller N, Paterson-Brown S. A prospective randomised controlled trial of the Kiwi Omnicup versus conventional ventouse cups for vacuum-assisted vaginal delivery. BJOG 2006;113(2):183–9.

31. Murphy DJ, Koh DK. Cohort study of the decision to delivery interval and neonatal outcome for emergency operative vaginal delivery. Am J Obstet Gynecol. 2007;196(2):145 e1–7.

# Chapter 3
# Non-technical Skills

Rachna Bahl and Bryony Strachan

---

## Key Learning Points

■ To define and explain the importance of non-technical skills in obstetric practice.

■ To describe the nontechnical skills useful when conducting assisted vaginal birth (AVB).

■ To describe examples of good behaviours.

---

*Well I guess when you think of forceps and ventouse ... it just sounds very scary and having your feet up in stirrups and just lying there not feeling anything ... having lots of people whizzing all around you, it is quite scary you sort of feel like 'a piece of meat on a butcher's table' in a way you do feel quite helpless because you just have to ... you're at the mercy of the doctors having to hope they're doing their best in a way.*

*A mother*

The components of a good AVB are complex and layered. They go far beyond a degree of knowledge and technical ability. They encompass a range of cognitive and social skills that promote respect for women and their partners and enable an environment in which women feel safe and secure, acknowledging her rite of passage and the privilege of assisting at the birth of a new life. This chapter explores our understanding of these important 'non-technical' skills of a consummate accoucheur.

# What Are Non-technical Skills?

Non-technical skills are cognitive, social and personal resource skills required in an operational task involving decision-making and teamwork.[1,2] These are distinct skills, separate from an obstetrician's knowledge of the instruments and the technique and manual dexterity. These skills or lack of them have been identified as contributors to a significant proportion of adverse events in health care.[2,3] A study of adverse events in surgery identified communication issues as the causal factor in 43% of errors made.[4]

Similar findings have been identified in obstetrics. A joint commission into the study of errors in obstetric care concluded that failures of teamwork and communication were the cause of 70% of adverse events.[5] Similar findings have been noted in more recent UK maternity reports. The Kirkup report, focusing on organisational failures in a maternity unit, cited lack of teamwork and poor interpersonal relationships as a contributory factor.[6] Each Baby Counts report from 2015 showed that human factors were contributory in 30% of cases with lack of situational awareness and stress and fatigue as the most frequent individual factors.[7] An in-depth analysis of 50 cases of compensation claims for cerebral palsy highlighted the value of timely decision-making.[8]

Non-technical skills have been studied in surgical, anaesthetic and acute medicine domains using methodology from the aviation industry.[9–12] Assisted vaginal birth (AVB) merits non-technical skills unique to this very intimate and emotive time for the mother and her birth partner. Unlike the scenarios studied in anaesthesia and surgery, the mother is awake and her cooperation and confidence in the caregivers can influence the outcome of the procedure. In the vast majority of cases, the decision to conduct an AVB is made in the second stage of labour when the mother is arguably at her most distressed and vulnerable. Assisted vaginal birth is considered a deviation from natural childbirth which the mother generally believes to be the utopian or ideal way of giving birth.[13] Assisted birth, dissatisfaction with antenatal care and the presence of unwanted personnel in the labour room have all been associated with a greater risk of postnatal depression among mothers.[14] Therefore, the obstetrician needs to be aware of not only the cognitive but also the social and interactive non-technical skills required when performing an AVB.

# Classification of Non-technical Skills

A three-tier behavioural system is used to classify non-technical skills.

The first level has six major categories of these skills.[9–11] When conducting an AVB, the main categories to be considered are:

- situational awareness
- decision-making
- teamwork and communication
- professional relationships with the woman
- maintaining professional behaviour
- dealing with stress and fatigue.

Each category is subdivided into elements. The elements define observable individual skills. For each element, identified examples of good behaviour are described.

Table 3.1 describes skills for an individual obstetrician rather than the multidisciplinary team. The reason for defining the skills for an individual is to enable each team member to be aware of his/her training needs in their domain. If all team members have good non-technical skills relevant to their area of expertise, the team is likely to function efficiently. Moreover, healthcare practitioners work in temporary teams and the team members change with every shift. Therefore, individual skills need to be addressed as well as the team's non-technical skills.

When describing non-technical skills for training, they are divided into three main groups:

- Cognitive skills such as situational awareness and decision-making. Good problem-solving, sound judgement and effective decision-making are considered among the highest attributes of clinicians.[15]
- Social skills such as teamworking, communication, maintaining professional behaviour and developing a professional relationship with the mother. These skills are not new to obstetricians, and experienced obstetricians have always demonstrated these skills as an integral part of their practice. However, it is important that trainee obstetricians are aware of these observable skills because they can have a significant impact on the physical and psychological outcomes of the AVB.
- Dealing with stress and fatigue such as reflection, developing resilience and seeking support from colleagues and friends.

**Table 3.1** Non-technical skills required for assisted vaginal birth

| Category | Element |
| --- | --- |
| **Cognitive skills** | |
| Situational awareness | Gather information |
| | Understand and analyse information |
| | Anticipate hazards |
| | Plan contingencies |
| Decision-making | Consider all options |
| | Implement one option |
| | Evaluate/reassess the option chosen |
| **Social skills** | |
| Teamwork and communication | Clear exchange of information |
| | Identify resources |
| | Be aware of team capabilities |
| | Have respect for members of the team |
| | Cross-check: be a 'wing man' |
| Professional relationship with the woman | Communicate with the mother |
| | Maintain respect for and ensure dignity of the mother |
| Maintaining professional behaviour | Partner participation |
| | Calm confident/assertive able |
| **Personal resource skills** | |
| Dealing with stress and fatigue | Reflection |
| | Resilience training |
| | Support from colleagues and friends |

# Categories of Non-technical Skills

## Situational Awareness

Situational awareness is defined as the perception of elements in the environment, comprehension of their meaning and the projection of their status in the near future.[16] It essentially means that the operator is aware of what is going on and how it can affect the outcome. The term 'situational awareness' was first used in the military and has since been used in the aviation industry. It was introduced to medicine in anaesthetics when crew resource management training used in aviation was used as a model for team training in anaesthesia.[17] A good pilot will be 'ahead of the plane' and have planned his/her route, acknowledging potential hazards such as weather patterns or an unusual airport approach or mechanical factors for which he/she has planned contingencies so that the flight is smooth and uneventful. Likewise, a good obstetrician will be 'ahead of the labour ward' and will have an up-to-date briefing of the labour ward board, anticipating which women may need obstetric help and when, will have an understanding of staffing matters and will have planned for contingencies. Situational awareness is an important skill in conducting a safe instrumental birth. Gathering appropriate information and assimilating it to make the decision that provides the best option for mother and baby is vital in minimising the morbidity associated with AVB. Situational awareness enables the obstetrician to make an appropriate decision when deciding whether an AVB is indicated and, if indicated, where it should be conducted and what should be the instrument of choice.

## Examples of Good Practice: Situational Awareness

### Information gathering:

- reviews the antenatal history and progress in labour
- reviews maternal and fetal well-being
- conducts abdominal and vaginal examination
- cross-checks information and checks the state of the labour ward.

### Understanding and analysing information:

- identifies risk factors predisposing to a need for AVB
- identifies factors that can help reduce the likelihood of AVB.

### Anticipation:

- implements factors to facilitate normal birth where applicable
- anticipates complexity of the planned AVB and takes relevant actions
- anticipates potential complications and has planned contingencies, for example for increased risk of failure to deliver or postpartum haemorrhage.

Various situational awareness strategies have been shown to reduce the likelihood of requiring an AVB in order to promote a spontaneous birth. Continuous support during labour, use of upright or lateral positions, avoiding epidural and delayed pushing in primiparous women with an epidural can reduce the need for an AVB. When called to review a mother with a view to conducting an AVB, in the absence of suspected fetal distress, certain strategies can be considered to avoid an AVB (Figure 3.1).

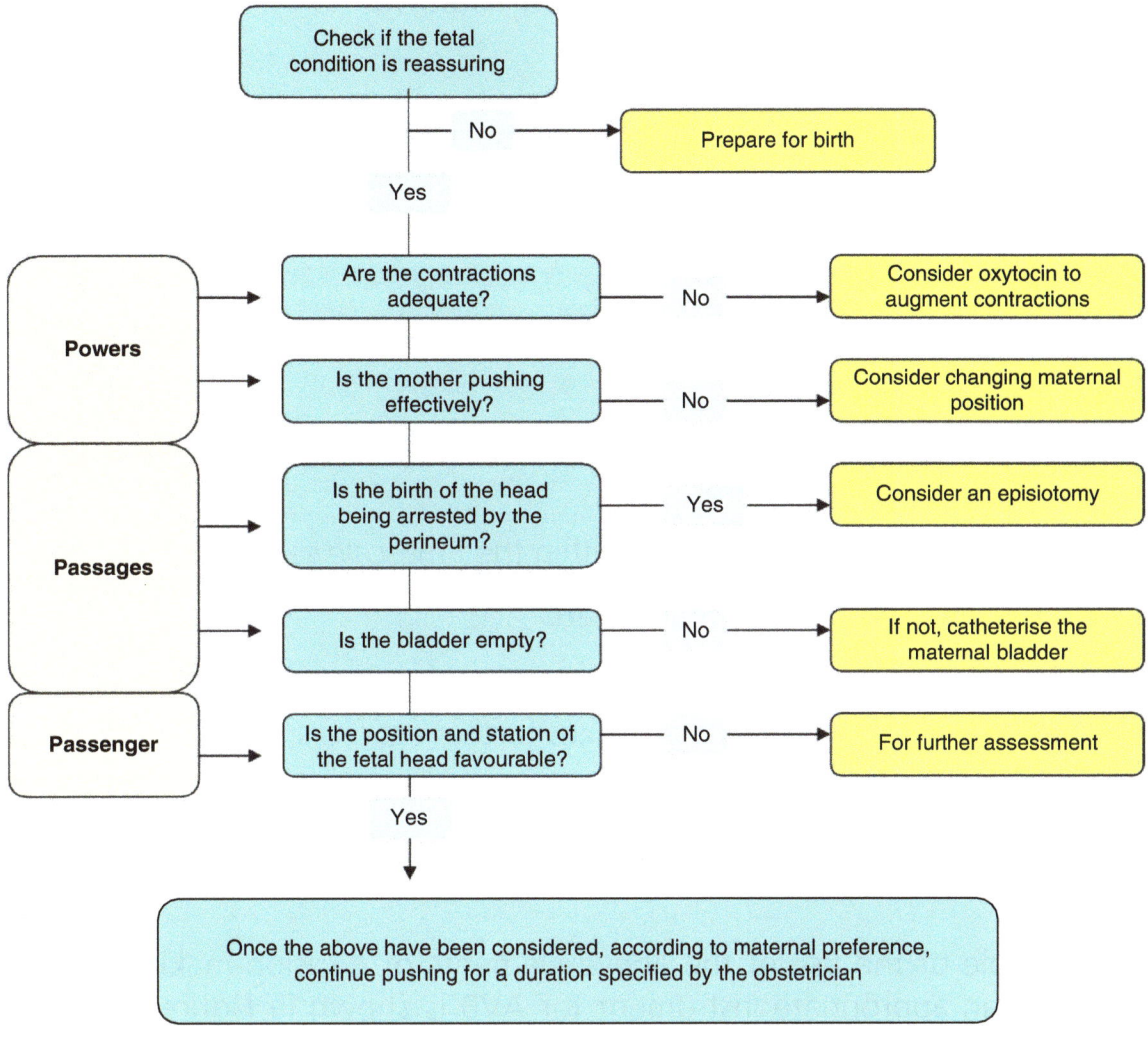

**Figure 3.1** Strategies to improve spontaneous birth.

## Decision-Making

Decision-making is the process of reaching a judgement or choosing an option to meet the needs of a given situation.[15] It is a cyclical process where an action is selected and continually re-evaluated. Any deviation from anticipated progression leads to a change in action to achieve the optimum result.

The behavioural markers for the three elements of the decision-making skill are shown below. Trainees should become familiar with these behavioural markers when training in simulation or when dealing with non-urgent clinical situations. Familiarity with the decision-making elements will enable obstetricians to implement these processes in stressful clinical situations and facilitate them to make appropriate decisions.

*Examples of Good Practice: Decision-Making*

**Consider all available options:**

- generates the options of whether to conduct the birth in the labour room or in the operating theatre in the context of the clinical situation
- generates the options of various instruments that can be used to conduct the birth
- discusses the options with the mother and her partner.

**Implement one option:**

- considers the risks and benefits of various options and selects the most appropriate option
- implements the selected option within the timescale selected.

**Evaluate/reassess the option chosen:**

- reviews the progress at each step
- if progress is not as anticipated, takes further actions such as:
  - ☐ call for senior support
  - ☐ change the course of AVB
  - ☐ abandon procedure.

An example of the use of the above elements of decision-making when selecting an appropriate instrument for AVB is shown in Figure 3.2. The obstetrician needs to consider the cues from situational awareness when making a decision about the most appropriate instrument for conducting the AVB. Once the instrument has been selected and the procedure has

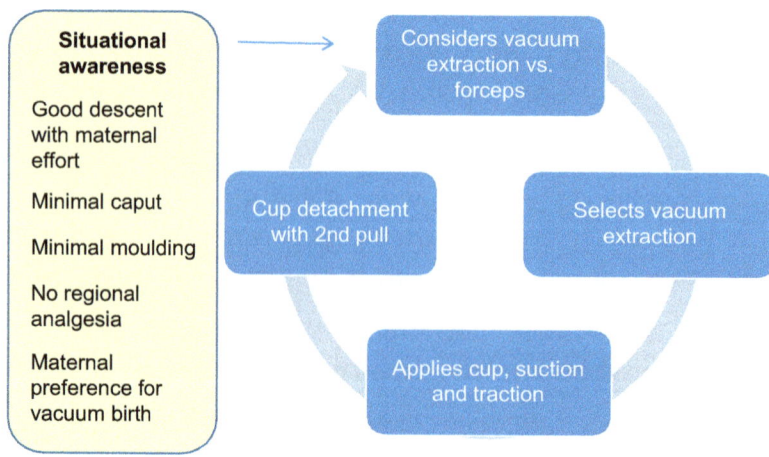

**Figure 3.2** Decision-making for selecting an appropriate instrument for AVB.

begun, it is important to reassess at each step. In the scenario detailed above, there were no deviations from the anticipated progress until the traction was applied for the second time. At this stage, the cup detached from the fetal scalp. This situation prompts the obstetrician to reassess the clinical situation. The decision regarding further action will be based on the most likely cause for cup detachment and the likelihood of achieving a vaginal birth.

## Teamwork and Communication

The most commonly known non-technical skills are teamwork and communication. Teamworking is the skill of working in a group of health professionals and ensuring that the efforts are directed at reaching the common goal. As a team worker, the focus is not only on the task but also on the team members.

Exchange of information is vital when co-ordinating the team to perform a task. This helps in gathering information (situational awareness) and selecting the most appropriate action (decision-making). Communication can be verbal or nonverbal, but it is important that the message being communicated is explicit and unambiguous. The purpose of the communication is that the message is received and understood by the team member it is directed at. Poor communication not only compromises team morale and safety, but it is also noticeable to the mother. It has been reported that poor communication between health professionals can lead to dissatisfaction with the care a mother receives during childbirth.[19] Once the decision for conducting an AVB has been made, the obstetrician should communicate clearly to the midwife looking after the mother and the midwife in charge of the labour ward.

One should be aware not only of one's own ability but also the capability of the team. Obstetricians are often aware of or make an effort to establish the ability of a trainee who they are supervising. However, it is also important to ensure that the midwife is aware of her/his role in this scenario and their role has been communicated to her/him clearly. If the midwife needs support, this should be identified and arranged. A good team is one in which the members support each other. If one is not aware of the limitations of the team members, it can often become difficult to limit harm done by the less able professional. All of us will need a support and a 'wing man' to look out for us at some time. One of the cornerstones of teamworking is that team members have mutual respect for each other. This holds true for the team working when conducting an AVB. It is important for team morale and performance that the team members are treated in a manner that makes them feel respected and valued. If a conflict arises, every effort should be made to resolve it instantly.

Below are the behavioural markers identified for obstetricians in the context of AVB.

## *Examples of Good Practice: Teamwork and Communication*

**Clear exchange of information:**

- informs the midwife caring for the woman of the urgency, instrument and the place of birth
- discusses with the midwife in charge of the labour ward and ensures that AVB is appropriately prioritised in relation to the workload on the labour ward.

**Identify resources:**

- ensures all the necessary equipment is available
- ensures that the instruments are available easily on the trolley
- ensures that all the personnel are present and ready for the birth
- delegates tasks clearly.

**Aware of team capabilities:**

- ensures that the midwife in the room understands her/his role
- ensures that the midwife is competent and confident about her/his role in the birth.

**Respect for team members:**

- is polite to the team members when asking for equipment
- registers and acknowledges their opinion
- debriefs and thanks team after a difficult birth.

## Professional Relationship with the Woman and Her Birthing Partner

This category does not feature in the taxonomy of surgical non-technical skills and is unique to obstetrics. During labour and birth the woman and her partner are aware of the proceedings in the room and anticipate full participation. In the study into non-technical skills of obstetricians conducting AVB, this category was considered extremely important by obstetricians and midwives. The elements that form this category arguably constitute the behaviours a woman is likely to remember, and these behaviours will have a great impact on her perception of the birth.

Communication with the mother is the main building block for developing a professional relationship with her. Communication is two-way and active listening to the mother and her partner at their most vulnerable time is vital.

## Professional Behaviour

Trust is a key component in any doctor-patient relationship. At assisted deliveries this is even more critical as women often have to relinquish their control and allow a stranger to make decisions about the well-being of their unborn baby. Trust in the doctor was reported as an important feeling. The qualities in doctors that instil trust are important to address and women described many good behaviours that had a positive impact on their experience. Calm, confident, caring, reassuring and assertive but not intimidating behaviour were common themes which made women feel they were in safe hands. Similarly, acknowledgement of the distress a woman may experience was an important behaviour. Women who felt that this was not recognised felt negatively towards their experience. Recognition that assisted delivery is not what women had planned, and thus may feel a sense of failure or disappointment, can be helpful to ease the transition from preformed plans to reality. Positive encouragement, assessment of well-being and handing back control back to the woman were good behaviours that were seen as positive by women.[18]

*Examples of Good Practice: Professional Relationship with the Woman*

**Communication with the mother:**

- introduces her/himself to the mother and her partner
- explains what her/his role is and why asked to review
- explains the proposed procedure clearly and in easy-to-understand terms
- asking about the mother's well-being
- explains the commonly anticipated complications
- listens to the mother's concerns and attempts to address them

- tailors care to the mother's wishes, such as preference for a particular instrument
- obtains informed consent
- keeping the woman in control.

**Maintain the dignity of the mother:**

- makes an effort to cover the mother
- keeps the door to the delivery room closed
- minimises unnecessary visits to the room
- asks and uses the mother's preferred name.

**Partner participation:**

- involves the birthing partner in the decision-making process.

## Maintaining Professional Behaviour

This category is considered a vital non-technical skill by obstetricians and midwives. The elements discussed here are described as key leadership skills when detailing non-technical skills in other domains. A team leader is defined as a person who is appointed, elected or informally chosen to direct or co-ordinate the work of others in a group.[19] However, during the study of non-technical skills of obstetricians conducting an AVB, it was felt that the above definition did not always apply to the obstetrician. The leader of the AVB is sometimes not the leader of the complete clinical situation. This becomes apparent when a junior trainee is conducting the AVB and a senior midwife is maintaining situational awareness and leadership of the whole clinical scenario. The clinical situation where the patient is actively involved throughout the procedure brings another dimension to this category. The boundary between assertiveness and aggressiveness is sometimes blurred when leading a task. However, with AVB, it is essential that the obstetrician is assertive but not aggressive towards the team or the mother. Therefore, the category is named 'maintaining professional behaviour'.

One of the common indications for AVB is suspected fetal compromise. This is an anxious time for the mother, and it is therefore essential that the obstetrician appears calm and in control. As the obstetrician is leading the team, his/her attitude will have an influence on how everyone else in the room perceives the situation. A junior trainee may not be confident about performing the procedure. The trainee should be aware of his/her limitations, but it is important that the lack of confidence is not apparent when conducting the birth. It is also important that the obstetrician appears able and assertive during the birth.

*Examples of Good Practice: Maintaining Professional Behaviour*

**Calm:**

- stays calm in an emergency situation
- does not appear stressed.

**Confident/assertive:**

- creates a confident atmosphere, provides clear, firm instructions and takes the lead.

**Able:**

- knows his/her limitations
- is open and honest about his/her ability and reflects on the experience
- is gentle and shows empathy.

## Dealing with Stress and Fatigue

Work-related events have been reported to lead to stress among obstetricians.[20] A national survey of obstetricians and gynaecologists in UK reported high levels of burn-out, more so among trainees.[21] These doctors are more likely to practise defensive medicine. Fatigue and stress have also been shown to be associated with medical errors.[22] Increasing fatigue can impair function leading to the detriment of other non-technical skills. It is important that obstetricians develop skills to deal with stress and fatigue. Reflecting on one's stress and fatigue levels is the first step to recognising and mitigating the likelihood of error. Effective feedback following a stressful event can have a benefit on performance.[23] Resilience training can help in dealing with stress and breaking the vicious circle of self-perceived medical errors and resultant poor self-esteem, emotional distress and burn-out.

*Examples of Good Practice: Dealing with Stress and Fatigue*

**Reflection:**

- aware of one's fatigue or stress
- seeks support if concerned about own performance
- analyses task after completion and seeks feedback.

**Resilience:**

- develops own strategies to cope with stressful situation.

**Support from colleagues and friends:**

- builds positive professional relationships
- formal or informal mentoring
- has good social network of support.

# Discussion

Assisted vaginal birth requires complex technical and non-technical skills. The decision-making processes become more challenging when the information is incomplete and the clinical situation highly emotive.[24,25] Decision aids can be used to reduce the relative effort needed for making a decision. Knowledge of the principles of situational awareness and explicit decision-making skills can aid trainees' understanding of when to intervene, where best to conduct the birth and the optimal choice of instrument for an AVB in relation to clinical assessment in the second stage of labour.

The social and interpersonal skills not only contribute to patient safety but also can lead to a lasting impression on the mother. Therefore, the value of these should not be under-estimated and need to be carefully built into teaching and formative assessments.

Classification of skills into categories and elements is helpful when developing a training package as well as to structure feedback to trainee obstetricians. Use of simulation and video feedback can be useful to discuss these skills with trainees. The limitation of this behavioural marker system is that it describes individual skills that are easy to observe and does not include every cognitive skill. We have focused on the observable skills because the main aim is to use the system for future training.

# References

1. Flin R, O'Connor P, Crichton M. *Safety at the Sharp End: A Guide to Non-technical Skills*.Boca Raton, FL, USA: Ashgate; 2008.

2. Bogner M. (editor). *Human Error in Medicine*. Hillsdale, NJ: LEA; 1994.

3. Bogner M. (editor). *Misadventures in Health Care*. Mahwah, NJ: LEA; 2004.

4. Wilson J. A practical guide to risk management in surgery; developing and planning. Healthcare Risk Resources International – Royal College of Surgeons Symposium 1999.

5. Guise JM, Segel S. Teamwork in obstetric critical care. Best Pract Res Clin Obstet Gynaecol 2008;22:937–51.

6. Kirkup DB. The Report of the Morecambe Bay Investigation. 2015.

7. RCOG. Each Baby Counts: 2015 Full Report. London; 2017.

8. Magro M. Five years of cerebral palsy claims: a thematic review of NHS Resolution data. London: NHS Resolution; 2017.

9. Flin R, Maran N. Identifying and training non-technical skills for teams in acute medicine. Qual Saf Health Care. 2004;13 Suppl 1: i80–4.

10. Fletcher G, Flin R, McGeorge P et al. Anaesthetists' Non-Technical Skills (ANTS): evaluation of a behavioural marker system. Br J Anaesth 2003;90:580–8.

11. Yule S, Flin R, Paterson-Brown S, Maran N, Rowley D. Development of a rating system for surgeons' non-technical skills. Med Educ 2006;40:1098–104.

12. McCulloch P, Mishra A, Handa A et al. The effects of aviation-style non-technical skills training on technical performance and outcome in the operating theatre. Qual Saf Health Care 2009;18:109–15.

13. Frost J. Pope C, Liebling R, Murphy D. Utopian theory and the discourse of natural birth. Social Theory & Health 2006;4:299–318.

14. Astbury J, Brown S, Lumley J, Small R. Birth events, birth experiences and social differences in postnatal depression. Aust J Public Health 1994;18:176–84.

15. Croskerry P. The theory and practice of clinical decision-making. *Can J Anaesth* 2005;52: R1–8.

16. Endsley M. Towards a theory of situational awareness in dynamic systems. Human Factors 1995;37:32–64.

17. Gaba D, Howard S, Small S. Situational awareness in anesthesiology. Human Factors. 1995;37:20–31.

18. Cass G, Goyder K, Strachan B, Bahl R. Can we improve women's experience of operative birth? European Journal of Obstetrics & Gynecology and Reproductive Biology. 2020. In press.

19. TNS for the COI Communications (on behalf of Department of Health). NHS Maternity Services Quantitative Research, The Stationery Office, October 2005. www.dh.gov.uk/assetRoot;?04/12/42/44/04/12422.pdf

20. Wahlberg Å, Andreen Sachs M, Johannesson K et al. Post-traumatic stress symptoms in Swedish obstetricians and midwives after severe obstetric events: a cross-sectional retrospective survey. *BJOG* 2017; 124: 1264–71.

21. Bourne T, Shah H, Falconieri N et al. Burnout, well-being and defensive medical practice among obstetricians and gynaecologists in the UK: cross-sectional survey study. BMJ Open 2019;9: 2019–030968.

22. Shanafelt TD, Balch CM, Bechamps Gerald MD[†§] et al. Burnout and medical errors among American surgeons. Annals of Surgery: 2010; Volume 25; Issue 6: 995–1000.

23. Hall LH, Johnson J, Watt I, Tsipa A, O'Connor DB. Healthcare Staff Wellbeing, Burnout, and Patient Safety: A Systematic Review. PLoS one 11(7): e0159015. https://doi.org/10.1371/journal .pone.0159015

24. Bowen J. Educational strategies to promote clinical diagnostic reasoning. N Engl J Med 2006;355:2217–25.

25. Charlin B, Boshuizen HP, Custers EJ, Feltovich PJ. Scripts and clinical reasoning. Med Educ 2007;41:1178–84.

# Chapter 4
# Vacuum-Assisted Birth

Glen L Mola, Stephen O'Brien and Aldo Vacca

---

## Key Learning Points

- Importance of the flexion point in vacuum-assisted birth and how to achieve correct cup application to the fetal head.
- Technique to reduce failure and cup detachment rates when performing vacuum-assisted birth.
- Technical aspects and good clinical practice points to improve the safety of vacuum-assisted birth for the mother and newborn.

---

When a valid indication for vacuum-assisted birth exists, the relevant obstetric variables should be identified and carefully assessed to determine whether vacuum-assisted birth is appropriate and safe under the clinical circumstances and for the level of experience of the operator. This important decision-making process is considered in Chapters 2 and 3 of the book. This chapter focuses on a few selected technical matters that should, if followed, improve the efficacy and reduce the risk of vacuum-assisted birth.

## Essential Principles for Vacuum-Assisted Birth

### The Flexion Point and Optimising Fetal Head Diameters to Maximise Success of Vacuum-Assisted Birth

The flexion point is a point on the sagittal suture of the fetal scalp, 3 cm anterior to (i.e. in front of) the posterior fontanelle.[1] It marks the exit point of the mentovertical diameter and is a critical landmark for vacuum-assisted birth. When the centre of a vacuum cup has been placed over the flexion point and axis traction is applied, the fetal head will flex with traction and head diameters will be optimal for birth. Regardless of the position of the head, the operator should be able to locate the flexion point and correctly position the cup over (or even posterior to) it (Figure 4.1). When a 5 cm cup is placed over the flexion point, the anterior rim of the cup will be at least 3 cm behind (i.e. posterior to) the anterior fontanelle. If a vacuum cup is placed more posterior (i.e. behind the flexion point), axial traction will still flex the head (Figure 4.2).

The midpoint of the fetal head is situated on the mentovertical diameter but within the cranium approximately 6 cm from the vertex. Its significance lies in the fact that the long axis of the fetal head pivots at the level of the midpoint as the head descends. Therefore, traction with a vacuum extractor should not be directed upwards until the midpoint has passed beneath the symphysis pubis. Furthermore, since the midpoint is situated at the same level as the widest diameters of the fetal head, the resistance to birth is greatest at this level and not at the level of the cup.

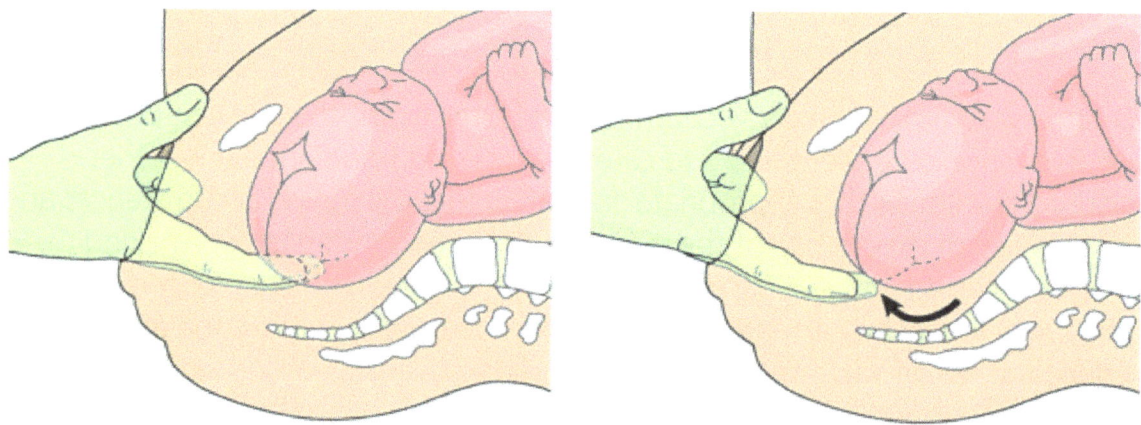

**Figure 4.1** Locating the flexion point.

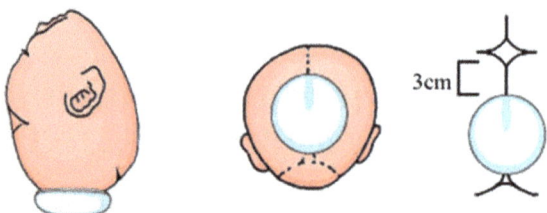

**Figure 4.2** The flexion point and cup relationships to fontanelles. To flex the head with traction, the cup must be at least 3 cm from the anterior fontanelle.

The implication for practice is that when the vacuum cup has reached the vaginal introitus, the widest diameters of the fetal head are still passing through the narrowest part of the birth canal, namely the pelvic floor and perineum. This phase of a vacuum-assisted birth is generally associated with higher resistance levels than those encountered during the descent phase.[2]

## Choice of Suitable Vacuum Cup

The design of a vacuum cup is the major factor that determines its manoeuvrability within the lower birth canal, and therefore its appropriate clinical use.[1] Manoeuvrability of a vacuum cup allows the operator to place the cup on the flexion point.

Vacuum cups that are commercially available include:

- Soft 'anterior' type cups (plastic or rubber):
  - ☐ Silc and silastic cups
  - ☐ Mystic MitySoft cup
  - ☐ Kiwi ProCup

- Rigid 'anterior' type cups (plastic or metal):
  - ☐ Malmström, Bird and O'Neil anterior cups
  - ☐ Kiwi OmniCup (anterior mode of cup placement and use)
  - ☐ M-Style Mystic Mityvac cup

- Rigid 'posterior' cups (plastic or metal):
  - ☐ Bird and O'Neil posterior cups
  - ☐ Kiwi OmniCup (posterior mode of cup placement and use)
  - ☐ h M-Select Mityvac cup

The rigid anterior cups (metal and plastic) and all soft cups are suitable (i.e. can be placed over the flexion point) if the occiput is anterior and the fetal station is low, or at the outlet. A posterior cup should be used for all occipito-transverse (OT) and occipito-posterior (OP) positions and for oblique anterior positions when the scalp is not visible between contractions.

Posterior cups are also the vacuum cup of choice for 'trials of vacuum extraction' (in theatre) and/or when attempting a mid-cavity extraction irrespective of the position of the occiput.

# The Five Steps of a Vacuum-Assisted Birth

## 1 Locating the Flexion Point and Calculating the Cup Insertion Distance

Before applying the cup to the fetal head, the position of the occiput is rechecked and the precise location of the flexion point is confirmed.[1] The cup insertion distance can then be estimated by using the middle finger of the examining hand (Figure 4.3). This calculation should be made during the vaginal examination conducted as part of the assessment of labour.

Generally, the insertion distance is approximately 5 cm (from posterior fourchette to the fetal head) for anterior positions of the occiput, 8 to 9 cm for transverse positions of the occiput and 10 to 11 cm for posterior positions. The Kiwi Omnicup has distances in centimetres marked on the traction tubing.

## 2 Holding and Inserting the Cup

The operator lightly smears the outside of the vacuum cup with obstetric cream and gently retracts the perineum with two fingers to form a space into which the cup is inserted with one movement immediately following a contraction. All rigid cups (both posterior and anterior cups) should be held with the thumb on the dome of the cup and two fingers on the rim nearest the operator. The soft cups are grasped near the broad flexible end and compressed to make insertion easier.

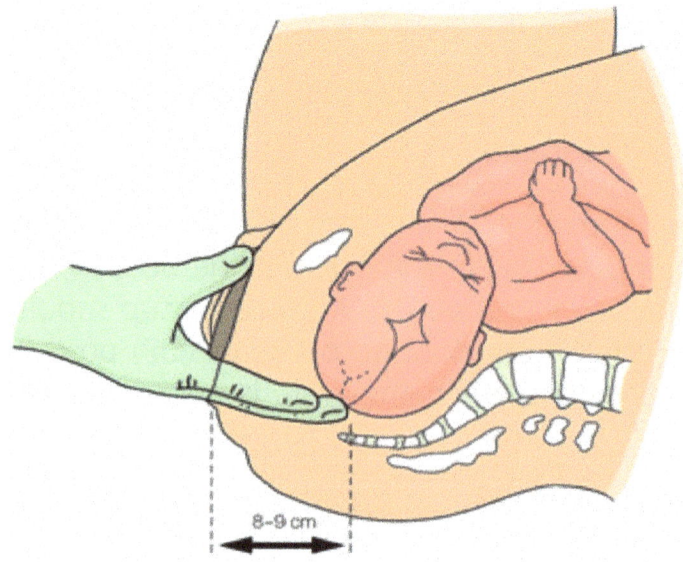

**Figure 4.3** Low OT, with asynclitism; digital and insertion distance 8–9 cm.

# 3 Manoeuvring the Cup Towards the Flexion Point

For low and outlet occipito-anterior (OA) positions, the flexion point will be located near the introitus. The cup should be placed 5 cm in and up under the fetal head (i.e. not on the presenting caput) and a little manoeuvring of the cup will be necessary to achieve a flexing median application. As stated above, the insertion distance is about 5 cm from cup to posterior fourchette. (This does not apply to operators using Silc cups as there is a long stem attached to the cup and the tubing is attached to this. The placement of a Silc cup over the flexion point relies upon the fetal head being low, anterior and flexed. Silc cups are not manoeuvrable once inserted into the introitus.)

The tissues of the labia minora and vestibule are in front of the fetal head. When vacuum-assisted delivery is being carried out at low and outlet stations, these may be at risk of entrapment beneath the vacuum cup. To avoid this problem, one hand holds the cup in position against the fetal head while the index finger of the other hand is swept around the periphery of the cup to exclude maternal tissue. This manoeuvre is not usually necessary when placing the cup for posterior and transverse positions of the occiput because the very act of pushing the cup up under the fetal head to the flexion point will push maternal tissues out the way.

For mid- and low-pelvic OP and OT positions, the flexion point will be displaced away from the introitus towards the sacrum and considerable manoeuvring of the cup will be required to achieve a correct application. Therefore, a manoeuvrable posterior-design cup should be selected for vacuum-assisted births where the fetal head is malpositioned. Displacement of the flexion point in both OP and OT positions is mainly in an anteroposterior direction of the birth canal and to a much lesser extent laterally. For practical purposes, therefore, the posterior cup should be manoeuvred in the mother's midline pelvic axis to the flexion point.[1]

Pushing a posterior cup up under the fetal head to the flexion point is best done between contractions and using the operator's two index fingers.

In OP and OT positions of the head it is usually not possible to reach the distal part of a correctly placed cup to exclude maternal tissue entrapment. In these cases the vagina is being pushed outwards by the widest diameters of the fetal head and insertion of the cup into the space between the head and pelvic floor will distend the vagina even further. For this reason, maternal entrapment under the cup is unlikely. Too vigorous an attempt to reach the distal parts of the cup may cause maternal discomfort or may dislodge the cup forwards away from the flexion point.

## 4 Inducing and Maintaining the Vacuum

Once the cup has been applied over the flexion point it should be held there with one index finger and the recommended vacuum pressure of 80 kPa may be attained in one step.[3] If the cup is not held at the flexion point while the vacuum pressure is applied, the cup has a tendency to slip forwards away from the flexion point. However, if the operator is not confident that the cup has been placed correctly, it is advisable to pause when a vacuum of 20 kPa has been reached to check the application and (with anterior position extractions) to exclude vaginal tissue entrapment.

Gentle traction may be started as soon as the next contraction begins and the mother begins to push. Stronger traction can be delayed for a period of time (about two minutes) to allow the chignon to form inside the cup. A practical tip is to apply the cup immediately after a contraction so that the chignon has some time to form before the next contraction begins.

Some operators reduce the vacuum to a lower level between contractions, although the evidence has not demonstrated any benefits for the fetus from this technique,[4] nor is there any evidence to support the view that levels of negative pressure below 80 kPa are associated with a reduction in scalp injury. For these reasons, it would seem preferable to maintain the vacuum at working levels until the head has been delivered.

## 5 Method of Traction

The operator should kneel on one knee or sit on a low stool so that traction can be applied in a downward direction along the axis of the pelvis. For low extractions when the scalp becomes visible or when the head has descended to the outlet, the direction of traction will change progressively, first in an outwards and then in an upwards direction. At this point, the standing position for the operator can become more appropriate.

Attachment of the cup to the scalp has been shown to be most effective when the direction of pull is perpendicular to the cup.[5] This is almost always possible during vacuum-assisted birth except in the initial stages in OP and OT positions when the head is deflexed or asynclitic. However, gentle downward traction will quickly correct the attitude of the head, after which perpendicular traction can be achieved.

In every instance it is important to apply traction perpendicular to a correctly applied cup, keeping the tube of the vacuum straight and without kinks.

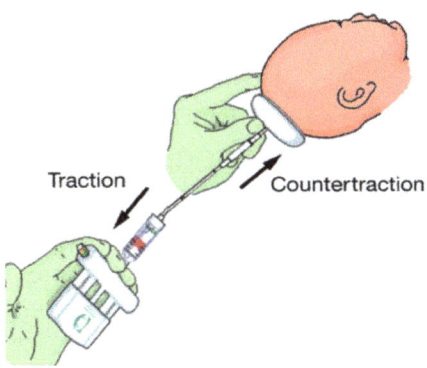

**Figure 4.4** The two-handed traction technique.

Traction should be performed as a two-handed exercise with both hands working in unison: one providing the traction (the 'pulling' hand) and the other monitoring the progress and providing counter-traction when necessary (the 'non-pulling' hand) (Figure 4.4).

Traction with the vacuum extractor should be regarded as an adjunct to the expulsive forces of labour and not as the primary means of overcoming tissue resistance to descent. If contractions are weak or infrequent, oxytocin infusion should be instituted promptly because the number, duration and strength of pulls required for birth are inversely proportional to the efficiency of the contractions and maternal effort and directly proportional to the adverse event rate once the number of pulls exceeds three.[2]

As a rule of thumb, the majority of instrumental deliveries for nulliparous women will benefit from second stage oxytocin augmentation, which is best set up as soon as the decision is made. This is particularly important for vacuum extraction, where good contractions and maternal expulsive efforts are a prerequisite for success.

## The 'Finger-Tip' Position of the Pulling Hand

Vacuum devices that are fitted with or incorporate a traction bar or handle should be held with the bar cradled in the slightly flexed distal interphalangeal joints with the palm of the hand opened and facing downwards (Figure 4.4).

The principal functions of the pulling hand are to direct traction along the axis of the pelvis so that the fetal presenting diameters are optimal for birth, that is, axis traction; to provide additional but not excessive traction to complement the mother's expulsive powers; and to pull only when the uterus is contracting and the mother is pushing.

## The 'Finger-Thumb' Position of the Non-pulling Hand

The standard position for the non-pulling hand should be with the thumb placed on the dome of the cup, providing some degree of counter-pressure when required during traction, and with the index finger of the same hand resting on the fetal scalp in front of the cup to monitor progress at the level of the midpoint of the head. Since most cup detachments occur when the cup is visible at the vaginal introitus, the finger-thumb position must be maintained until the head has crowned or delivered to reduce the risk of detachment.

Therefore, when perineal support (guarding) is practised, this should be provided by an assistant and not by the operator.

The principal functions of the non-pulling hand are to monitor progress with each pull – descent, flexion and autorotation – of the fetal head; to control the traction force transmitted to the fetal scalp by varying the amount of counter-pressure with the thumb; to avoid complete detachment ('pop off') of the cup by counter-pressure with the thumb; and being ready to provide counter-pressure during the perineal phase of delivery (the usual time for completion of autorotation to occur) and slowing progress across the perineum.

Axial traction with the vacuum extractor should result in progressive descent of the head with the least amount of traction force. Rocking movements from side to side or manually turning the rigid handles of some cups is contra-indicated because the shearing force or torque associated with such practices may increase the predisposition for cup detachment and fetal scalp injury.

Traction should commence at the onset of a contraction with the mother bearing down and should be maintained as long as she is pushing. The operator (and/or an assistant) should offer encouragement to the mother and inform her of the progress she is making. Usually women will manage two to three pushes per contraction. The operator should cease pulling when the woman stops pushing and recommence traction when she resumes expulsive efforts. As soon as the contraction passes, or the mother stops pushing, traction should be ceased.

Traction should not be continued between contractions; traction to 'maintain station' during the interval to prevent retraction of the head should not be applied because the force on the head, without maternal propulsive effort, may injure the fetal scalp or the mother's pelvic floor. Descent achieved at the end of one contraction will always be quickly regained at the start of the next contraction.

During the procedure, the fetal heart should be monitored regularly by continuous external electronic monitoring (or in some settings, by an assistant using a handheld device following each contraction).

# The Descent Phase and the Pelvic Floor Phase of a Vacuum-Assisted Birth

It is advisable to consider vacuum-assisted birth as a two-phase procedure: a descent phase and a pelvic floor/perineal phase.[2] The descent phase is that part of the vacuum extraction from application of the cup until the cup has descended to and is completely visible in the vaginal introitus. This marks the start of the pelvic floor phase, which lasts until completion of the delivery of the fetal head. In a prospective study of vacuum-assisted birth in nulliparous women, higher levels of traction force and a greater number of pulls were recorded in the majority of cases during the pelvic floor and perineal phase than during the descent phase.[2] An explanation for this may be that during the pelvic floor phase the widest diameters of the fetal head are negotiating the narrowest part of the maternal birth canal, and soft tissue resistance is maximal for the perineal phase of the birth, particularly in primigravidae.

# Signs of Progress

Operators should expect some progress to occur with each and every pull. Signs of progress are descent of the presenting part confirmed by the non-pulling hand, as well as flexion and correction of asynclitism and autorotation of the head in malpositions. When the head is deflexed or asynclitic, the first observed sign is usually flexion. This is evidenced by a visible increase in length of the tube or traction cord outside the vagina. Autorotation will be observed to some degree at all levels as the head descends. The head, not just the scalp, must begin to move with the first pull and some descent should occur with each subsequent pull.

Tractions that do not cause the head to descend ('negative' tractions)[6] must be differentiated from those that do, as they are more likely to cause subgaleal haemorrhage. Placing a limit on the number of pulls has been a principal safety measure recommended for avoiding injury to the newborn infant. For this reason, the concept of the 'three pulls rule' was introduced in 1964.[7] The rule states that 'If there is not good progress after the third pull, the case should be carefully reassessed.' When the rule was proposed, there were no epidurals, mothers were not pushing for long periods in the second stage and episiotomies were performed more liberally. Changes that have occurred in these obstetric practices over more recent times have important implications for vacuum-assisted birth. For this reason, the authors concur with the RCOG and recommend allowing three pulls for the descent phase and three pulls for the pelvic floor and perineal phase.[8] However, if the fetal head has not reached the pelvic floor by the third pull, the operator should reassess the situation and be confident of success before attempting a fourth pull.[1] For the avoidance of doubt, delivery should be 'imminent' after the third pull. Even though three further pulls might still be allowed for the perineal phase, 'imminent' in practical terms means that the presenting part is 'visible' between contractions without parting the labia and has started distending the perineum. Being able to see the tip of the caput whilst parting the labia at the peak of a contraction does not qualify for being either 'visible' or 'imminent'.

# After the Birth of the Head

After the birth of the head, the vacuum is released and the birth is completed in the normal manner. Sweeping a finger around the rim of the cup is useful for releasing the vacuum – the cup should never be pulled directly before the vacuum is released first.

Operators should always forewarn the parents prior to removal of the cup, and ideally before application, at the time of consent, about the appearance of the chignon and reassure them that the swelling will resolve quickly, and any marking caused by the cup will disappear completely.

As soon as possible after the birth the operator should palpate the area over the chignon with the fingertips to exclude possible subgaleal bleeding. This is particularly important if the birth was difficult or associated with cup detachment or minimal or no progress has occurred with any of the tractions. A fluid 'thrill' will be palpable under the cup application site if the scalp has been separated from the underlying cranium. Bleeding from damaged blood vessels when the scalp has been torn from the cranium will result in a subgaleal haematoma. The neonatal paediatric team should be informed of any concerns, especially if difficulty was experienced during the extraction, so that regular inspections of the scalp will be made. In this way, subgaleal bleeding will be detected early, allowing prompt and effective blood volume replacement (usually by IV or intraosseus 0.9% sodium chloride) to be instigated. As a rough rule of thumb, normal saline resuscitation should be in the usual ratio of 3:1: that is three times as much IV saline stat. as estimated volume of subgaleal haemorrhage. If a subgaleal haemorrhage is detected at birth then it is important to gain intravenous access before the baby becomes shocked making cannulation more difficult. A common mistake is to assume that neonatal shock is due to birth asphyxia and focus on ventilatory assistance alone.

On the day after the birth, the operator should re-examine the baby in the mother's presence to answer questions she may wish to ask and to allay any concerns she may express about the baby or the birth. In addition, it is an opportune time to discuss the reasons for the procedure and any other aspects that may require consideration in a subsequent pregnancy. Details of the procedure and the maternal and fetal outcomes should be accurately described in an assisted vaginal birth form designed to record relevant data about the procedure and to facilitate regular clinical audit.[8]

# Rotational Vacuum-Assisted Birth

Provided the operator has been adequately trained in the use of a posterior cup, the technique of rotational vacuum-assisted birth is identical to the five-step method described for non-rotational vacuum-assisted birth.[1] The complexity of a rotational vacuum procedure arises not from the technique itself but from the clinical circumstances associated with these procedures.

Anterior rotation of the malpositioned fetal head during vacuum extraction occurs automatically as a passive event similar to the internal rotation that is part of the mechanism of normal labour.

No attempt should be made to manually rotate the head either by manipulating the cup or by grasping a rigid handle and physically rotating the device.

An important but little appreciated fact in vacuum-assisted birth is the relationship between correct cup placement and autorotation of the fetal head. It has been demonstrated that autorotation rates of 90% or better can be achieved with vacuum extractions undertaken for OP and OT positions of the head provided there is a flexing application of the cup and traction that generates flexion.[9]

# Difficulty, Cup Detachment and Failure to Achieve Birth of the Fetal Head

Detachment of the cup may occur for one or more of the following reasons:

- deflexing or paramedian cup applications
- incorrect traction technique; pulling too hard, in the wrong direction or with a rocking motion

- not providing counter-pressure on the cup with the thumb during traction
- upwards traction before the midpoint of the head has passed beneath the pubic arch
- not allowing sufficient time for the perineum to stretch over the advancing fetal head, especially if episiotomy is not performed
- not appreciating that vacuum pressure has been lost, or heeding the suction noise (hiss) of loss of vacuum due to cup lift
- inadequate vacuum pressure, kinking of the tubing or faulty equipment.

Traction should be discontinued between contractions. If an audible 'hiss' is heard, signalling loss of vacuum and imminent cup detachment ('pop off'), traction should be stopped, and the vacuum pressure restored before the next traction. Incorrect application of the cup (deflexing or paramedian), pulling too hard and pulling in the wrong direction are common causes of cup detachment. Sudden cup detachment may injure the scalp, and should not be merely regarded as a safety mechanism of the vacuum extractor.[6] High detachment rates may reflect either problems with the instrument or with the way the instrument is used. The detached cup should be reapplied only if the operator is convinced that the cause of the detachment is not cephalopelvic disproportion. If detachment recurs or if the head fails to descend with traction in the descent phase, the procedure should be abandoned, and the birth completed by caesarean section.

Only if the detachment occurs during the perineal phase, with the vertex clearly visible in between contractions, should the delivery then be completed with forceps.

Most cup detachments occur when the cup is visible at or passing through the vaginal introitus. At this stage, the widest diameters of the fetal head, situated some six or seven centimetres behind the cup, are at the level of the mother's resistant pelvic floor and stronger traction may result in a cup detachment. Cup detachment may be prevented if the operator controls the rate of progress of the head across the perineum with thumb counter-pressure on the cup to give the perineum time to stretch over the advancing head. Upwards traction before the midpoint has passed beneath the symphysis pubis is another common cause of cup detachment. Placing a limit on the number of detachments has been recommended as a safety measure to protect the fetus against serious injury.

Most authorities accept three cup detachments as the upper limit.[8,10–13] However, it is advisable to consider every cup detachment as an event which needs to be analysed for reason and circumstances. If a cup detachment has occurred because of excessive pulling when there has been no clear progress, then the delivery attempt should be abandoned after that first detachment and with no more applications. However, if detachments are occurring because of a faulty instrument (e.g. blood clots are blocking the Kiwi cup tubing or tubing port in the cup), then it would be appropriate to continue the procedure with a new device.

Studies comparing vacuum extraction and forceps birth have consistently shown that the vacuum extractor is less likely than forceps to complete the birth.[14] A number of predisposing factors have been linked to failed vacuum extractions with or without cup detachment. They include (mostly clinically unrecognised) mid-cavity procedures, inadvertent deflexing and paramedian applications of the cup, use of soft cups in preference to rigid cups, extractions attempted before full dilatation of the cervix, cephalopelvic disproportion, and OP and OT positions of the head.[6,8,14] Indeed, one of the reasons that the vacuum extractor can cause suboptimal outcomes is the ease of application of the cup to the fetal head. With forceps it is generally not possible to correctly place the blades functionally on the fetal head when it is mid-cavity, when the cervix is not fully dilated or with pelvic curve type forceps in OP and OT positions of the occiput.

Inadequate (low frequency, short duration) contractions in nulliparous women can also impede success with vacuum extraction.

Malposition of the occiput should not be associated with failure per se. Indeed, correctable factors (like malposition or deflexion) should indicate that the procedure is more likely to be successful, as long as the operator is able to apply a posterior cup to the flexion point, and then flex the baby's head with traction. It is an anterior position where the fetal head is already fully flexed that is more likely to fail, for the reason that there is nothing that is 'correctable' by the instrument.

Failure of vacuum extraction with sequential use of forceps to complete the birth has been associated with increased risk of injury to the fetus[15,16] and to the maternal genital tract, relative to successful vacuum alone.[16,17] However, balanced against this is the significant, and often greater, maternal and neonatal trauma sustained from a second stage caesarean section, particularly when the head is low in the pelvis.[8] Moreover, in the two largest RCTs of different forms of vacuum, the overall failure rate was 24.7% (148/598), of which 117 (80%) were subsequently delivered with forceps, with no clinically significant injuries reported.[18,19]

This suggests that incorrect vacuum technique may have been a factor in a number of the births, and that most of the failures occurred at the outlet of the pelvis. The findings of this study should not be an excuse to use sequential instruments for a failed mid-cavity delivery after several attempts with minimal or no progress.

# Effects on the Newborn Infant

It is useful for counselling and auditing purposes to classify the effects of vacuum-assisted birth on the newborn infant in terms of their severity and clinical significance. A suggested classification is presented here:

■ cosmetic effects:

    ☐ the chignon (artificial caput succedaneum)

    ☐ cup discoloration and marking of the scalp

■ clinically non-significant injuries:

    ☐ blisters and superficial scalp abrasions

    ☐ cephalhaematoma[1]

    ☐ retinal haemorrhage

■ clinically significant injuries:

    ☐ extensive scalp lacerations

    ☐ subgaleal (subaponeurotic) haemorrhage

    ☐ intracranial haemorrhage

    ☐ skull fracture

■ indirect and coincidental injuries:

    ☐ brachial plexus injury

    ☐ fracture of the clavicle or humerus.

The current Cochrane Systematic Review[14] demonstrates that soft cups caused fewer scalp lacerations (29.9% versus 40.6%) and cephalhaematoma (8.15% versus 14.2%) than rigid cups. However, these effects are transient and do not pose threats to the well-being of the infant. The review did not however show a difference in clinically significant subgaleal or intracranial haemorrhages. Similarly, when neonatal outcomes of vacuum extraction and forceps birth were

---

[1] Cephalhaematoma is due to bleeding under the peri-osteum of the parietal bone. This is caused by friction between the fetal head and the side wall of the pelvis. The vacuum extractor does not in itself predispose to this injury and indeed cephalhaematomas occur in association with spontaneous vaginal birth. They are more common with forceps delivery because of the placement of the forceps over the parietal bones. They may be more common with vacuum extraction than with normal birth because of the fact that the head is being drawn through the pelvis and there is some tightness of fit leading to more friction forces on the side of the head.

compared in the review, differences were confined to the clinically non-significant effects.[14]

Subgaleal haemorrhage may be associated with a number of factors that are a feature of difficult vacuum-assisted births, including deflexing and paramedian cup applications, prolonged extractions with excessive number and strength of pulls (particularly when there has been no progress with any of the tractions), cup detachment (often multiple), and failure of the initial vacuum extraction with a subsequent attempt at forceps birth.[20,21]

# Effects on the Mother

Maternal perineal trauma causes both short- and long-term problems for women – in the short term, women can sustain obstetric anal sphincter injuries (OASI), faecal incontinence (FI), anal incontinence (AI), urinary incontinence (UI) and pelvic organ prolapse (POP) in the medium or long term.

These outcomes have significant impacts on maternal quality of life and future reproductive career. Taken together, women sustaining some degree of perineal trauma are more likely to report bothersome symptoms of urinary incontinence, faecal incontinence or pelvic organ prolapse from one year after birth[22] to 20 years after birth.[23,24] Moreover, women who sustained an OASI, compared to women who had a vaginal birth without OASI, are specifically more likely to report higher rates of faecal and anal incontinence,[25] and poorer sexual function,[26] as well as poorer overall quality of life overall.[27]

Importantly, vacuum-assisted birth is associated with lower rates of OASI than forceps birth – the most recent Cochrane meta-analysis reported OASI rates for all types of pooled forceps births of 14%, compared to 7.5% for all ventouse procedures.[14] This is supported by retrospective studies of national registries in the UK and the Netherlands, which have demonstrated two to three-fold higher rates of OASI among women delivered with forceps versus women delivered with ventouse.[28,29]

Therefore, unless operators are appropriately trained in vacuum extraction techniques to be able to complete the birth using vacuum when possible, and not resort to the use of forceps, the potential advantages for the mother's pelvic floor and perineum from vacuum births may not be fully realised.

The role of episiotomy in reducing maternal morbidity associated with vacuum-assisted birth is unclear. The only prospective study into the role of episiotomy at reducing OASI in instrumental birth did not show an association between liberal and restrictive use of episiotomy for vacuum-assisted births.[30]

Moreover, systematic reviews of observational studies of vacuum-assisted births show a non-significant association between use of episiotomy and a reduction in OASI in primiparous women (RR 0.68, 95% CI 0.43 – 1.07), but a statistically significant relationship between episiotomy and OASI in parous women (RR 1.27, 95% CI 1.05–1.53).[31,32]

However, a large UK-based registry study of 1.2 million nulliparous births demonstrated a reduction in the rate of OASI in vacuum births where episiotomy was performed compared to those in which it was not (RR 1.89, 95% CI 1.74–2.05).[29]

Pragmatically, for vacuum-assisted birth, episiotomy is not routinely required, but should be seriously considered at least in nulliparous women. For this reason, we advise infiltration of the perineum with local anaesthetic before commencing a vacuum extraction when the woman does not have an epidural. For outlet deliveries, local anaesthetic should still be strongly considered if the urgency allows. When performed, the episiotomy should be mediolateral rather than midline.[8,10]

# Conclusion

Vacuum-assisted birth and its acceptance by individual clinicians will be determined to a large extent by the number of successful births achieved and by the outcomes for the mother and infant. Clinical audits and system analyses often identify deficient knowledge and inadequate operator training as important contributors to adverse outcomes.[8,33,34] The key to avoiding suboptimal outcomes with vacuum-assisted birth is to ensure that the operator's knowledge, skill level and competence are equal to the requirements of the clinical circumstances.[33,35] Training programmes are now available that teach the technique on models that can simulate a realistic vacuum extraction procedure, and they should be undertaken by all obstetric trainees as part of AVB training.[8]

# References

1.  Vacca A. *Handbook of Vacuum Delivery on Obstetric Practice*. 3rd ed. Brisbane: Vacca Research; 2009.

2.  Vacca A. Vacuum-assisted delivery: an analysis of traction force and maternal and neonatal outcomes. Aust N Z J Obstet Gynaecol. 2006;46(2):124–7.

3.  Suwannachat B, Laopaiboon M, Tonmat S et al. Rapid versus stepwise application of negative pressure in vacuum extraction-assisted vaginal delivery: a multicentre randomised controlled non-inferiority trial. BJOG. 2011;118(10):1247–52.

4.  Bofill J, Rust OA, Schorr SJ, Brown RC. A randomized trial of two vacuum extraction techniques. Obstet Gynecol. No longer published by Elsevier; 19971;89(5):758–62.

5.  Muise KL, Duchon MA, Brown RH. Effect of angular traction on the performance of modern vacuum extractors. Am J Obstet Gynecol. 1992;167(4):1125–9.

6.  Bird GC. The use of the vacuum extractor. Clin Obstet Gynaecol. 1982;9(3):641–61.

7.  Lasbrey AH, Orchard CD, Crichton D. A study of the relative merits and scope for vacuum extraction as opposed to forceps delivery. SAMJ. 1964;38(3).

8.  Murphy DJ, Strachan BK, Bahl R. Royal College of Obstetricians and Gynaecologists. Assisted Vaginal Birth: Green-Top Guideline No. 26. BJOG. 2020 .

9.  Bird GC. The importance of flexion in vacuum extractor delivery. BJOG. John Wiley & Sons, Ltd; 1976;83(3):194–200.

10. ACOG. ACOG Practice Bulletin No. 154: Operative Vaginal Delivery. New York: ACOG; 2015:1–10.

11. Vayssière C, Beucher G, Dupuis O et al. Instrumental delivery: clinical practice guidelines from the French College of Gynaecologists and Obstetricians. Eur J Obstet Gynecol Reprod Biol. 2011;159(1):43–8.

12. RANZCOG. Instrumental vaginal birth. RANZCOG; 2015:1–25.

13. Society of Obstetricians and Gynaecologists of Canada. Guidelines for operative vaginal birth. Number 148, May 2004. Int J Gynaecol Obstet. 2005;88(2):229–36.

14. O'Mahony F, Hofmeyer GJ, Menon V. Choice of instruments for assisted vaginal delivery. O'Mahony F, editor. Cochrane Database Syst Rev. Chichester, UK: John Wiley & Sons, Ltd; 2010;(11):CD005455.

15. Towner D, Castro MA, Eby-Wilkens E, Gilbert WM. Effect of mode of delivery in nulliparous women on neonatal intracranial injury. N Engl J Med. 1999;341(23):1709–14.

16. Gardella C, Taylor M, Benedetti T, Hitti J, Critchlow C. The effect of sequential use of vacuum and forceps for assisted vaginal delivery on neonatal and maternal outcomes. Am J Obstet Gynecol. 2001;185(4):896–902.

17. Demissie K, Rhoads GG, Smulian JC et al. Operative vaginal delivery and neonatal and infant adverse outcomes: population based retrospective analysis. BMJ. British Medical Journal Publishing Group; 2004;329(7456):24–9.

18. Attilakos G, Sibanda T, Winter C, Johnson N, Draycott T. A randomised controlled trial of a new handheld vacuum extraction device. BJOG. Blackwell Science Ltd; 2005;112(11):1510–5.

19. Groom KM, Jones BA, Miller N, Paterson-Brown SA. A prospective randomised controlled trial of the Kiwi Omnicup versus conventional ventouse cups for vacuum-assisted vaginal delivery. BJOG. 2006;113(2):183–9.

20. Fortune PM, Thomas RM. Sub-aponeurotic haemorrhage: a rare but life-threatening neonatal complication associated with ventouse delivery. BJOG. 1999;106(8):868–70.

21. Chadwick LM, Pemberton PJ, Kurinczuk JJ. Neonatal subgaleal haematoma: associated risk factors, complications and outcome. J Paediatr Child Health. 1996;32(3):228–32.

22. Lipschuetz M, Cohen SM, Liebergall-Wischnitzer M et al. Degree of bother from pelvic floor dysfunction in women one year after first delivery. Eur J Obstet Gynecol Reprod Biol. 2015;191:90–4.

23. Gyhagen M, Bullarbo M, Nielsen TF, Milsom I. A comparison of the long-term consequences of vaginal delivery versus caesarean section on the prevalence, severity and bothersomeness of urinary incontinence subtypes: a national cohort study in primiparous women. BJOG. 2013;120(12):1548–55.

24. Gyhagen M, Bullarbo M, Nielsen TF, Milsom I. Faecal incontinence 20 years after one birth: a comparison between vaginal delivery and caesarean section. Int Urogynecol J. 1st ed. 2014;25(10):1411–8.

25. Salim R, Peretz H, Molnar R, et al. Long-term outcome of obstetric anal sphincter injury repaired by experienced obstetricians. Int J Gynaecol Obstet. 2014;126(2):130–5.

26. Palm A, Israelsson L, Bolin M, Danielsson I. Symptoms after obstetric sphincter injuries have little effect on quality of life. Acta Obst Gyne Scand. 2013;92(1):109–15.

27. Samarasekera DN, Bekhit MT, Wright Y et al. Long-term anal continence and quality of life following postpartum anal sphincter injury. Colorectal Dis. 2008 ;10(8):793–9.

28. Bavel J, Hukkelhoven CWPM, Vries C et al. The effectiveness of mediolateral episiotomy in preventing obstetric anal sphincter injuries during operative vaginal delivery: a ten-year analysis of a national registry. Int Urogynecol J.; 2017;29(3):1–7.

29. Gurol-Urganci I, Cromwell DA, Edozien LC et al. Third- and fourth-degree perineal tears among primiparous women in England between 2000 and 2012: time trends and risk factors. BJOG. 2013;120(12):1516–25.

30. Macleod M, Strachan B, Bahl R et al. A prospective cohort study of maternal and neonatal morbidity in relation to use of episiotomy at operative vaginal delivery. BJOG. 2008;115(13):1688–94.

31. Sagi-Dain L, Sagi S. Morbidity associated with episiotomy in vacuum delivery: a systematic review and meta-analysis. BJOG. 2015 ;122(8):1073–81.

32. Lund NS, Persson LKG, Jangö H, Gommesen D, Westergaard HB. Episiotomy in vacuum-assisted delivery affects the risk of obstetric anal sphincter injury: a systematic review and meta-analysis. Eur J Obstet Gynecol Reprod Biol. 2016;207:193–9.

33. Hotton E, O'Brien S, Draycott TJ. Skills training for operative vaginal birth. Best Practice & Research Clinical Obstetrics & Gynaecology. 2019;56:11–22.

34. Reid HE, Hayes D, Wittkowski A et al. The effect of senior obstetric presence on maternal and neonatal outcomes in UK NHS maternity units: a systematic review and meta-analysis. BJOG. 2017;124(9):1321–30.

35. Bahl R, Murphy DJ, Strachan B. Qualitative analysis by interviews and video recordings to establish the components of a skilled rotational forceps delivery. Eur J Obstet Gynecol Reprod Biol. Elsevier; 2013;170(2):341–7.

# Tribute to Dr Aldo Vacca (1941–2014), Author of the Chapter on Vacuum-Assisted Delivery in the First Edition of the RoBUST Manual – by Glen Liddell Mola

Aldo Vacca became interested in vacuum-assisted delivery as registrar to Dr Geoff Bird at the Port Moresby General Hospital, Papua New Guinea in the 1970s when Dr Bird was doing the original research on the physics and mechanics of how the vacuum extractor can optimise assisted delivery by application of the vacuum cup to the 'flexion point' on the fetal head. In 1976 Dr Bird developed the 'posterior cup' from this research, which was the first vacuum cup that allowed the accoucheur to apply the vacuum cup to the flexion point in posterior and transverse positions of the occiput (even when the fetal head is deflexed). Dr Vacca was the lead researcher in the landmark RCT of vacuum and forceps at Portsmouth hospital in 1981–82 (BJOG, 1983) which clearly showed that 'Maternal trauma, use of analgesia and blood loss at delivery were significantly less in the group allocated to vacuum extraction.' This RCT was an important driver leading to the fact that today the vacuum extractor is the instrument most commonly used for assisted vaginal delivery in the UK. In the 1990s Dr Vacca worked with engineer Dr Dean Wallace of Clinical Innovations Inc., USA to develop a disposable plastic handheld vacuum device (the Kiwi omnicup – which is one of the commonest vacuum devices in use in the world today), as well as a reusable version called the 'Vacca re-useable ominicup'. (Aldo derived no financial gain from any of these device developments.) Dr Aldo Vacca spent the last 18 years of his professional life (1995–2013) touring the world providing hands-on vacuum-assisted delivery training in countries as diverse as Italy, Russia and India; he regularly attended the RANZCOG, RCOG and ACOG annual scientific meetings and offered day workshops for doctors (and midwives) wishing to upgrade their assisted vaginal delivery skills using a very lifelike pelvic model (Lucy and Lucy's Mum) which he developed in conjunction with ModelMed Ltd in Melbourne, Australia. In the UK Dr Vacca was a regular visitor to St George's Hospital, University of London (and some other hospital labour wards) where he would conduct week-long hands-on AVB training on 16-hour shifts in the delivery suite. To quote from the obituary by Professor Sir Sabaratnam Arulkumaran (BMJ, 2014), 'Aldo Vacca will be remembered as a legend in the obstetric world; as an excellent clinician, teacher, researcher, and medical leader par excellence.'

# Chapter 5
# Non-Rotational forceps and Manual Rotation

Kim Hinshaw and Shilpa Mahadasu

## Key Learning Points

- Developing skills in non-rotational forceps and manual rotation remain an important element of training in operative obstetrics.

- Informing women in the antenatal period about the frequency and methods of assisted vaginal delivery is a priority.

- Use simulation training to develop appropriate skills.

- Forceps are more likely to achieve vaginal birth compared to vacuum extraction but are associated with a higher risk of vaginal and perineal trauma.

- Forceps should be applied with care, and correct application to the fetal head should be confirmed before traction is applied.

- Initial traction should be applied using Pajot's manoeuvre, keeping the forceps handles near the horizontal plane until the fetal head is crowning.

- As the occiput passes under the symphysis pubis, elevate the forceps handles early, cease active pushing, slow down the delivery and maintain manual perineal protection.

- The operator must maintain situational awareness, review whether progress is adequate and be willing to seek help and abandon the procedure if necessary.

- Reassess and discuss with senior staff before proceeding with 'double instrumentation'.

- After forceps birth, always undertake a systematic inspection to exclude maternal trauma.

- Ensure comprehensive record keeping and debrief the mother after birth.

Assisted vaginal birth (AVB) is to expedite birth for the benefit of the mother, baby or both whilst minimising maternal and neonatal morbidity. Forceps, ventouse (or 'vacuum') delivery and manual rotation (usually completed with non-rotational forceps) are the most common methods used in the UK. In the UK, operative delivery rates have varied between 10 and 15%[1] (England 12.7% and Scotland 12.1% – data for 2021)[2,3] but rates vary significantly across European countries (median 7.2%; range 2.1% [Slovakia] to 15.1% [Ireland and Spain] – data for 2015).[4]

An updated Cochrane review of 31 studies (*n* = 5,754) compared forceps and vacuum delivery.[6] Forceps delivery are less likely than vacuum *to fail to achieve vaginal birth*: risk ratio (RR) 0.58, 95% confidence interval (CI) 0.39–0.88; [11 studies, 3,080 women; low certainty]. *'Any maternal trauma'* was more likely with forceps: odds ratio (OR) 1.53, 95% CI 0.98–2.40; [5 studies, 1,356 women; low certainty]. Third- or fourth-degree tears were more likely with forceps: RR 1.83, 95% CI 1.32–2.55; [9 studies, 2,493 women; low certainty], but there was no difference in the incidence of postpartum haemorrhage (PPH): RR 1.71, 95% CI 0.59–4.95; [2 studies, 523 women; low certainty]. Neonatal morbidity was similar in terms of low Apgar score and low umbilical artery pH, but with lower rates of fetal trauma with 'any forceps' for cephalhaematoma, retinal haemorrhage or jaundice.

The aim of clinical training is to ensure that we produce obstetricians who are aware of the circumstance in which a particular instrument should be used and who develop appropriate skills in the various techniques of AVB. This will ensure that we offer women a safe and effective assisted birth.

# Non-rotational Forceps

Non-rotational forceps are mainly used to facilitate vaginal birth when the fetal head is in an occipito-anterior (OA) position. Ideally, the fetal head will lie in the direct OA (DOA) position, but blades can be safely applied when the head lies within 45 degrees of the vertical (i.e. between left OA and right OA positions [Figure 5.1]). Non-rotational forceps may also be used to assist birth in a direct occipito-posterior (DOP) position.

The basic design constitutes a matching pair of forceps blades, with nominated left and right relative to where the blade lies when applied within the maternal pelvis. The relevant parts of the forceps are labelled in Figure 5.2 (a & b).

Several types of forcep are in common use in the UK, but all are essentially similar in configuration – long-handled types: Simpson, Anderson, Haig-Ferguson, Neville-Barnes; short-handled type: Wrigley's. The choice of forceps

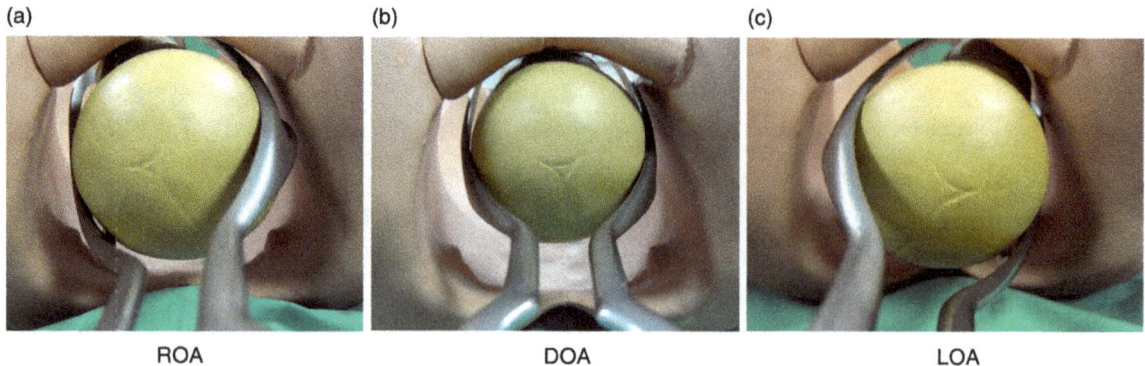

| (a) | (b) | (c) |
| --- | --- | --- |
| ROA | DOA | LOA |

**Figure 5.1** Range of positions for safe forceps application.

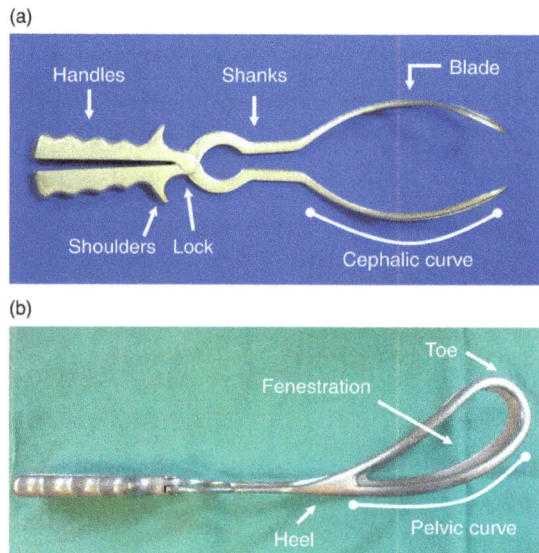

**Figure 5.2** Parts of the forceps.

is based on individual circumstances and is often subjective and based on preference in a particular unit or region. The majority of non-rotational forceps have relatively long handles allowing their use from mid-cavity level. Wrigley's forceps have short shanks and handles and are used to assist birth of the head at caesarean section or as outlet forceps in AVB (Figure 5.3).

# Assessment before Performing Non-rotational Forceps

Before embarking on a forceps delivery, remember that safe assisted vaginal birth requires careful assessment of the clinical situation, clear communication with the woman, her partner and supporting healthcare personnel, as well as

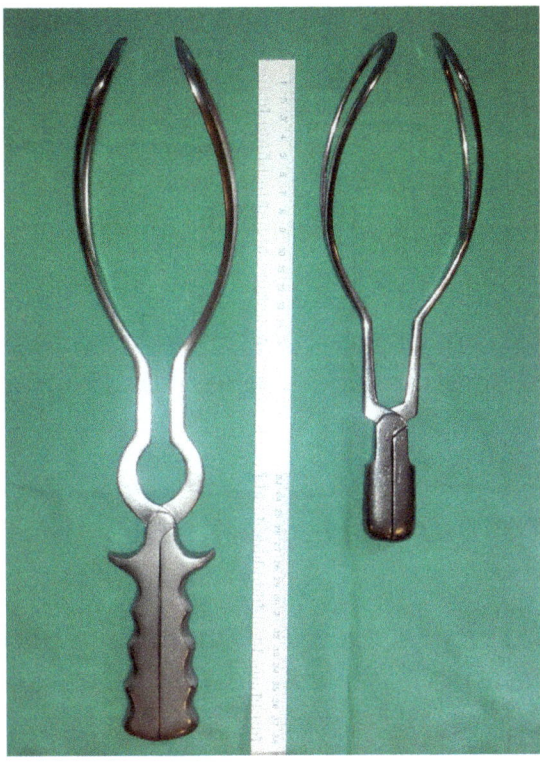

**Figure 5.3** Long- and short-handled forceps.

expertise in the chosen procedure.[1] Clear communication should occur before, during and after the procedure (including an appropriate debrief). Shared decision-making, along with good communication, and positive continuous support during labour and delivery can reduce psychological morbidity following birth.[1]

## Indications

The indications for considering AVB are discussed in depth in Chapter 2. The most common reasons for AVB are a prolonged second stage and presumed fetal compromise. Operators should be aware that no indication is absolute and that clinical judgement is required in all situations.[1] In the majority of cases, whether for maternal or fetal reasons, the choice between forceps and vacuum depends on the experience of the operator and their assessment of the best instrument to use *in the individual circumstance*.

Non-rotational forceps should be used and vacuum avoided in certain circumstances:

- face presentation (mento-anterior position)
- assisted birth under 32 weeks.[1]

Non-rotational forceps may be considered in preference to vacuum:

- in acute fetal compromise (prolonged bradycardia)
- for assisted birth at 32–36 weeks[1]
- for mid-cavity birth OA (particularly a trial in theatre)
- following *multiple* attempts at fetal scalp sampling.

Suspected fetal bleeding disorders or a predisposition to fracture (e.g. osteogenesis imperfecta) are relative contraindications to assisted vaginal birth, when an individualised decision about mode of birth has to be made by a senior obstetrician.[1]

## Clinical and Ultrasound Assessment

Assessment before undertaking an AVB is discussed in depth in Chapter 2. Careful abdominal and vaginal examination must be performed before undertaking a non-rotational forceps birth. Clinical examination should include consideration of any degree of relative (or absolute) disproportion. A common reason for clinical negligence litigation is failure to assess the position/level of the fetal head in relation to the pelvic outlet. Most cases of assisted birth where the position is OA are low cavity. Clinical assessment should start with a comprehensive abdominal examination. Assessment of position is usually made using the fontanelles and sutures as landmarks. In cases of significant caput, the operator can seek out the pinna of the fetal ear.

## Consent

Providing information about AVB for women in the antenatal period, especially during their first pregnancy, should facilitate the consent process in labour. Information on AVB from the RCOG Patient Information Committee is available online.[10] This is particularly important after the 2015 Montgomery determination which has clarified UK law and set new standards for consent.[11] Doctors have a duty to ensure that patients understand the material risks of any medical intervention and the risks of any reasonable alternatives. However, it is important to note that the 'material risks' are those *that the patient feels are relevant,* and no longer only those issues that medical staff feel are relevant.

For birth room procedures, verbal consent should be obtained prior to assisted vaginal birth and the discussion should be documented in the notes.[1] If circumstances allow, written consent may be obtained. Concerns to be covered include the proposed procedure, intended benefits, serious and frequently occurring risks both maternal and fetal (e.g. forceps marks on the baby's face), other procedures that may be required (for forceps birth, episiotomy should be mentioned) and planned analgesia/anaesthesia.[12,13]

Revised RCOG guidance recommends that when mid-pelvic (or rotational) birth is indicated, the risks and benefits of assisted vaginal birth should be compared with the risks and benefits of second stage caesarean birth, for the given circumstances and skills of the operator. Written consent should be obtained for a trial of assisted vaginal birth in theatre.[1] Consent for assisted vaginal delivery is now more complex and all obstetricians should ensure that they are familiar with the approach to consent that is required.[14] An example consent form is available as an appendix in the RCOG operative vaginal delivery consent advice document.[12]

# Technique for Non-rotational Forceps

## Preparation

Before embarking on a non-rotational forceps birth, the operator should be comfortable and competent to use the selected forceps with the ability to manage any complications that may arise. Adequate senior supervision must be available and present if required.[1] Skills lists are available that clearly delineate the steps required to achieve a safe AVB.[15] Again, remember that clear communication with the woman, her partner and the rest of the maternity team is vital, before, during and after the procedure.[1] Having obtained appropriate consent from the woman, the operator should ensure that the following factors are also addressed:

- **Team**: A complete team should be available to support the operator. This will vary but may include midwives, a healthcare assistant, a professional trained in neonatal resuscitation, an anaesthetist and senior obstetric staff.
- **Analgesia**: Ensure effective analgesia is given. Options for forceps include pudendal block, perineal infiltration, regional blockade and, rarely, general anaesthesia (see Chapter 9).
- **Check instruments**: Check that all necessary equipment is laid out on the trolley in the correct order. Three clamps (two for dividing the cord and one for clamping the cord for cord bloods) and scissors for performing an episiotomy if required. Count all swabs before proceeding and ensure that this is recorded.
- **Positioning**: A modified lithotomy position is best, avoiding excessive hip abduction. The mother should be supported in a semi-upright position and, where possible, some degree of (left) lateral tilt should be maintained. The buttocks should just protrude beyond the end of the bed.

■ **Positioning of the operator**: Operators vary in their preference to sit, stand or kneel while conducting a forceps birth. The operator should be well balanced, predominantly using hands and arms only to apply traction force. Sitting or kneeling may reduce the temptation to use (potentially excessive) upper bodyweight during traction.

■ **Catheterisation**: The operator should gown and glove up appropriately for the procedure before cleansing and draping. The bladder should normally be emptied using an 'in and out' catheter. Occasionally this is not possible if the head is very low near the pelvic outlet. If an indwelling catheter is present, it should be removed prior to proceeding with the assisted delivery (it can be replaced afterwards).

■ **Confirm clinical findings**: Before applying the forceps blades, recheck presentation, position, level, etc.

## Forceps Application

■ **Check that the forceps are a *matching* pair**: all forceps have a number imprinted on them and these should match. Also ensure that the blades fit easily together and lock appropriately.

■ **Assembly**: place the forceps on the trolley 'back-to-back' with the toe of each blade pointing upwards. Pick up the left blade with the left hand and right blade with the right hand (Figure 5.4a). To assemble the forceps, the blades are crossed, with the right blade lying superior to the left (Figure 5.4b). They meet and join at the 'lock' (Figure 5.4c).

■ **Applying the left blade**: the left blade is inserted first. Do not hold the forceps by wrapping all four fingers around the handle, as this may encourage use of inappropriate force during insertion. The handle should be held in a vertical position between the thumb and the index and middle fingers of the *left* hand, using a 'light pencil grip' (Figure 5.5a). This grip reminds the operator to avoid using excessive force during insertion. The index and middle fingers of the *right* hand are inserted through the introitus at the 'five o'clock' position and the tip of the left blade is introduced to lie just within the introitus. Keep the handle vertical and parallel to the patient's *right* femur, with the inner surface of the forceps blade initially facing the presenting part of the fetal head. The fingers of the right hand are moved laterally to protect the maternal soft tissues, and the blade is gently inserted to lie in the final position against the left side of the fetal head, parallel to the sagittal suture. This requires the blade to be gently rotated through 90 degrees (along its long axis) as it is inserted. The thumb of the right hand can be placed on the heel of the blade to help insertion. After insertion, the handle is pushed gently back against the perineum to help hold the blade in position (Figure 5.5a–c).

(a)

(b)

(c)

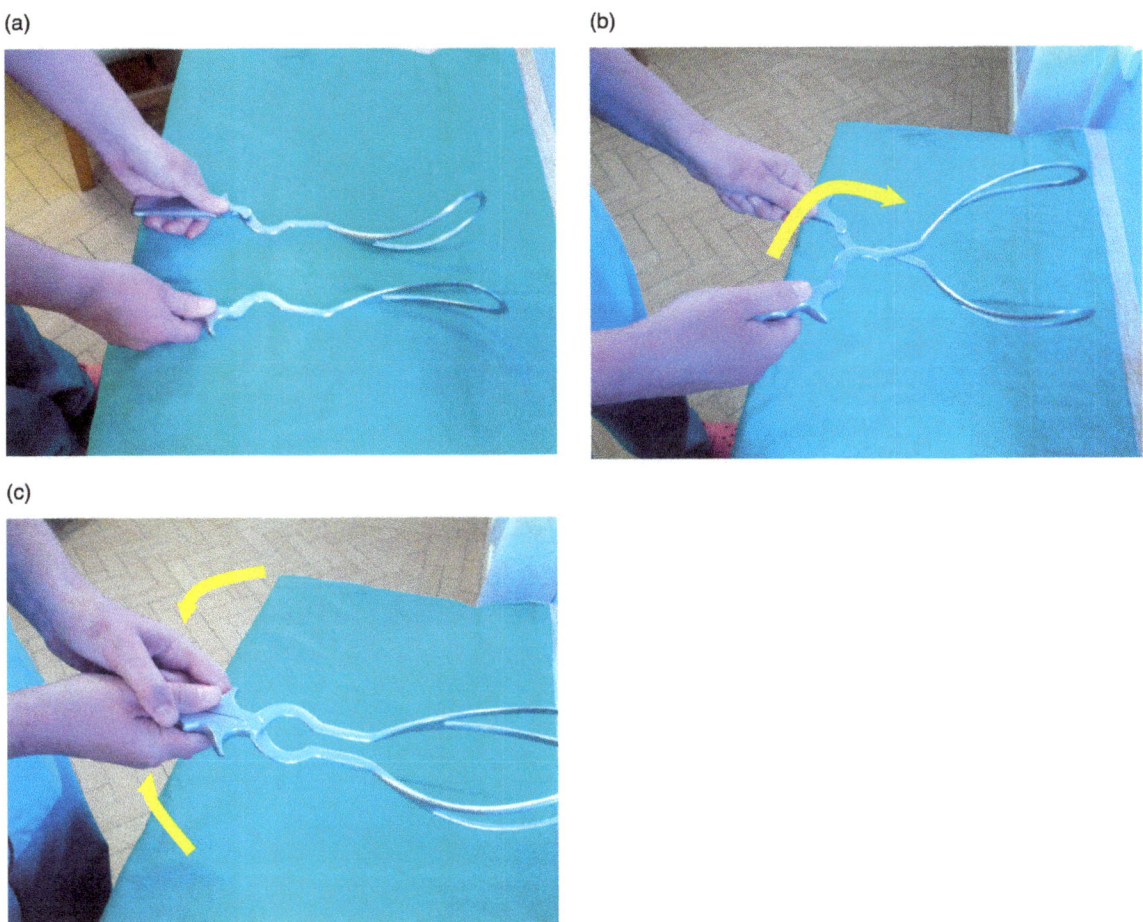

**Figure 5.4** Assembling the forceps.

Change hands for insertion of the right blade. The right blade is held vertically with the right hand using the same light pencil grip. The index and middle fingers of the left hand are inserted through the introitus at the 'seven o'clock' position, using the same technique as described for the left blade. Insertion of both blades should occur easily (Figure 5.6a–c). If insertion proves difficult, remove the blade(s) and carefully recheck the position of the head. Call senior staff if you're unsure.

- **Locking the blades**: the left blade is always inserted first, allowing the two forceps blades to be locked without having to 'uncross' the handles. After insertion, the blades will need gentle manipulation in order to get them to 'lock' (Figure 5.7a and 5.7b). Once locked, the operator should avoid holding the handles together as this may compress the fetal head.

- **Confirming correct application**: before applying traction, the operator should check that the blades are correctly applied to the fetal head (Figure 5.8a and 5.8b). Run the tip of an index finger along the shanks of the forceps to confirm good application:

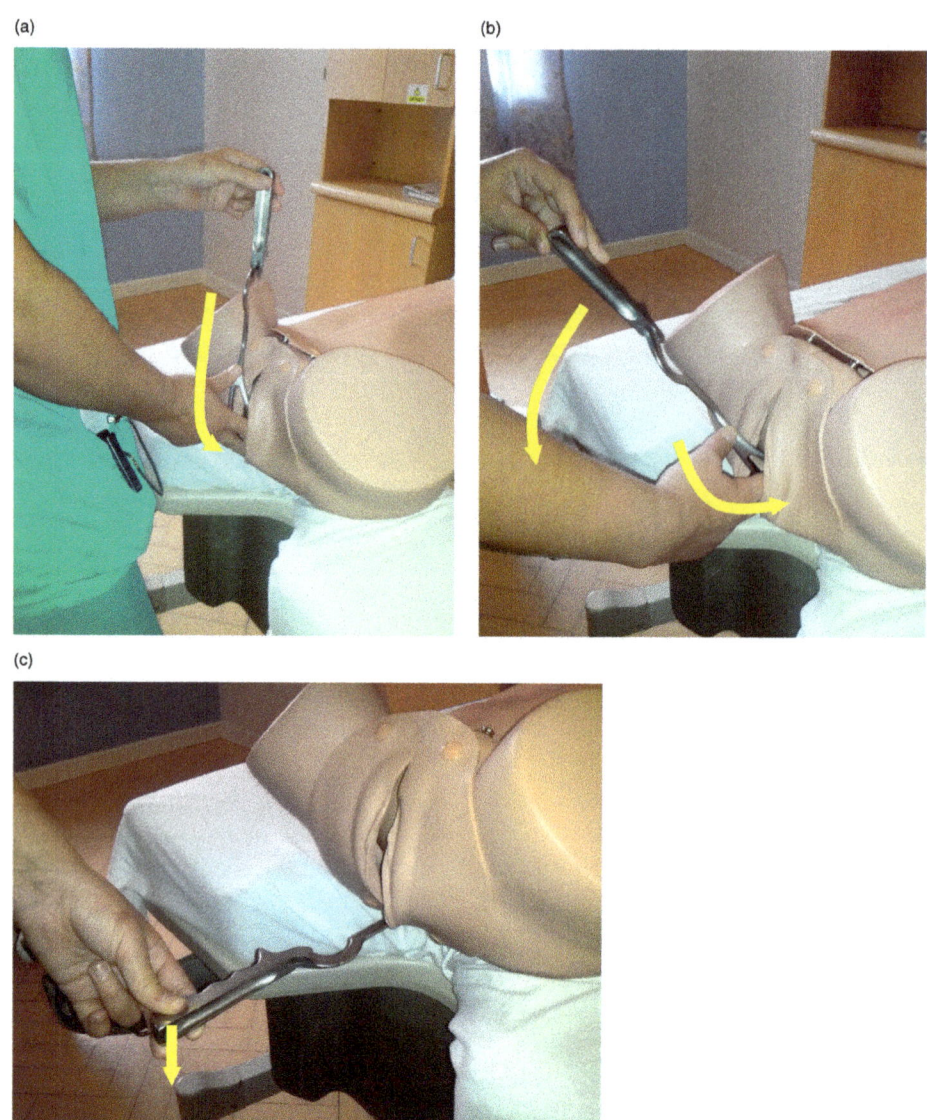

**Figure 5.5** Applying the left blade.

☐ the sagittal suture should be central between the blades and lie parallel to the plane of the blades

☐ in the OA position, the lambdoidal sutures should be equidistant from the upper edge of both blades

☐ the posterior fontanelle should be no more than 1–2 cm above the level of the shanks

☐ it should not be possible to introduce more than a fingertip through the fenestration near the heel of the blade (i.e. from 'inside to out').

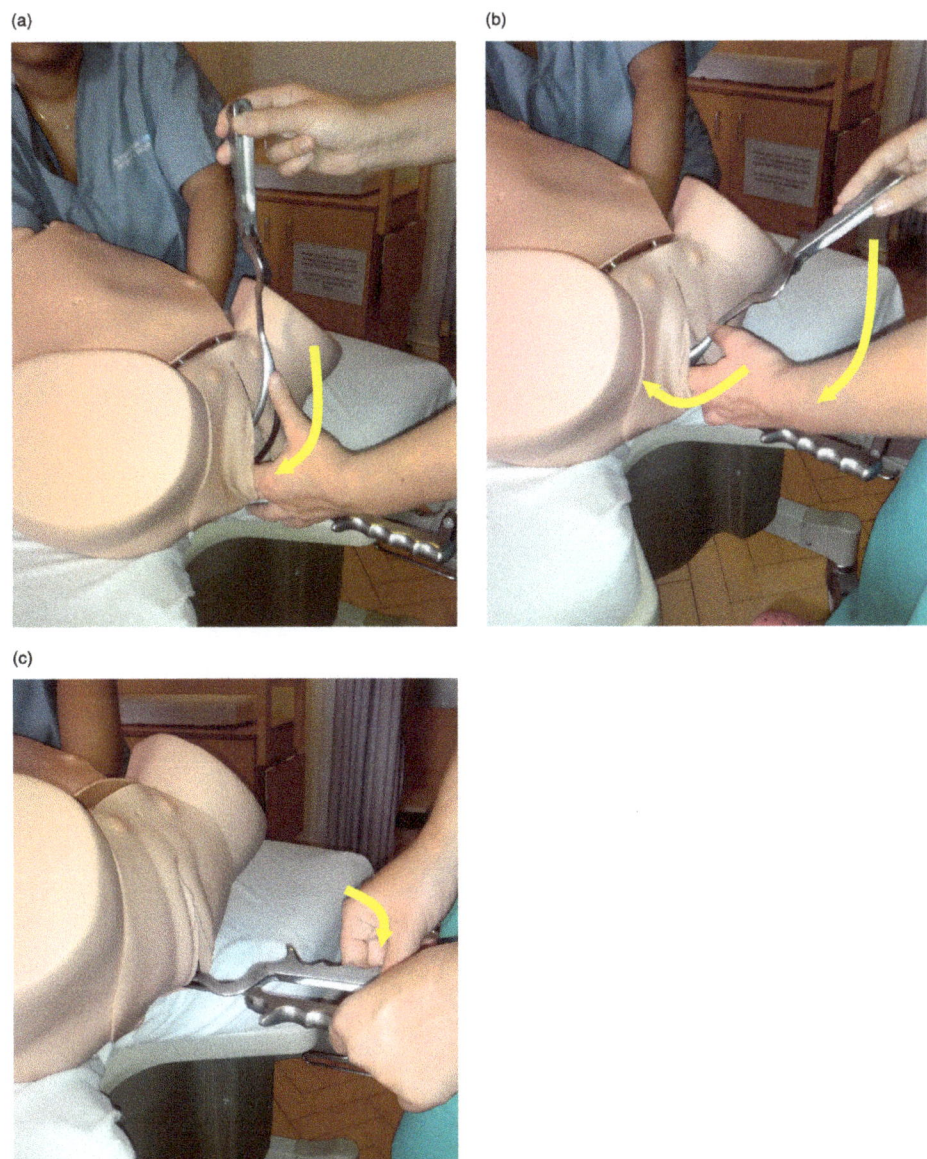

**Figure 5.6** Applying the right blade.

When the head is OA and well flexed, a well-applied forceps blade should lie along the mento-vertical axis of the fetal skull (Figure 5.9). Traction force is mainly applied to the fetal malar bones, accounting for the pressure mark that is often found at that point immediately after birth.

## ■ Application of the blades in LOA or ROA position:

Non-rotational forceps can be applied and used in a safe range, 45 degrees either side of the maternal sagittal plane (Figure 5.1). With an LOA or ROA position, the

(a)                                    (b)

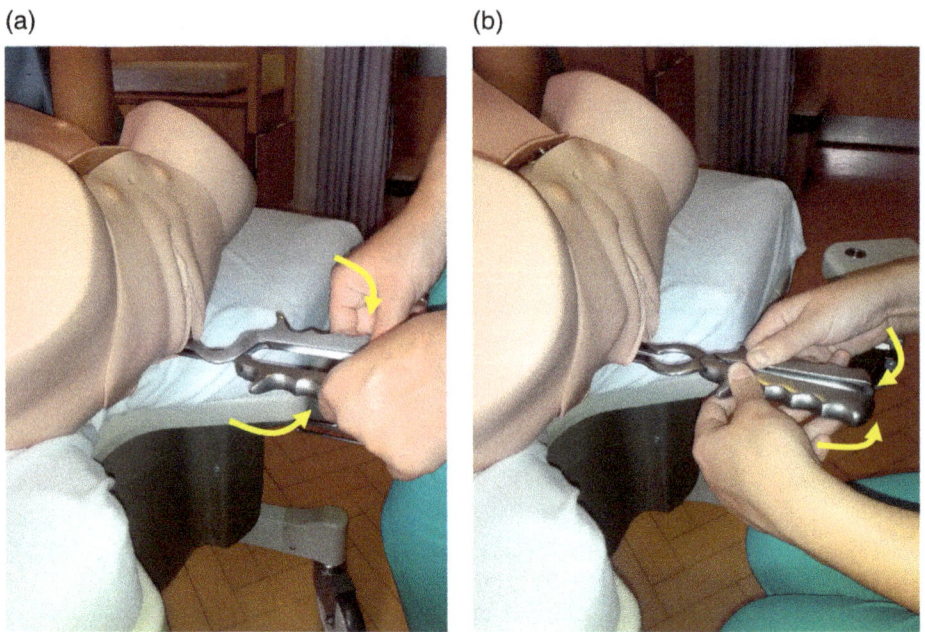

**Figure 5.7** Locking the blades.

(a)                    (b)

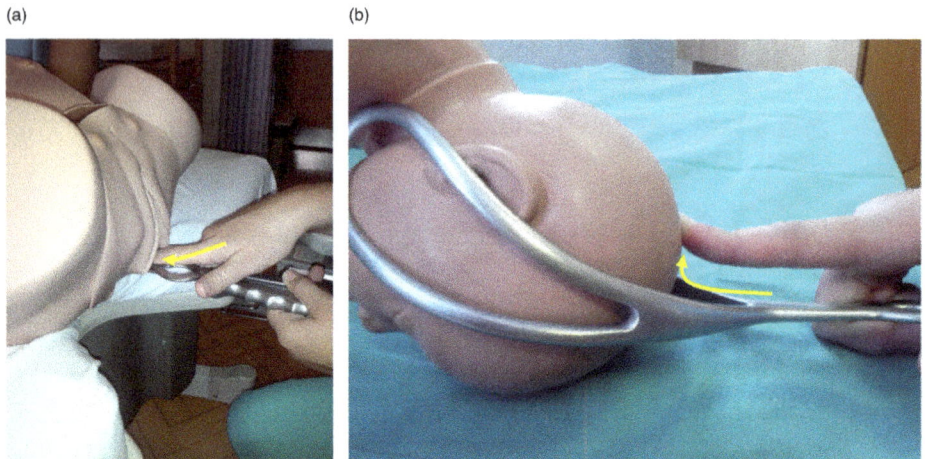

**Figure 5.8** Confirming correct application.

insertion procedure is essentially the same, but care must be taken to ensure that appropriate rotation of each blade occurs along its long axis. This will ensure that both blades *lie parallel to the sagittal suture*. [Remember – the sagittal suture will be rotated away from the vertical plane in LOA or ROA positions (Figure 5.1).]

Before applying traction, rotation from ROA/LOA to the 'direct OA' position is easily achieved. Elevate the handles gently upwards and outwards:

i. in the LOA position this means elevating the handles towards '1 to 2 o'clock'
ii. in the ROA position towards '10 to 11 o'clock'.

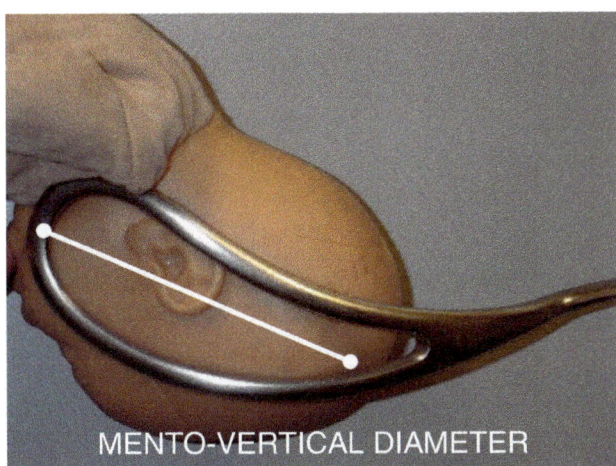

MENTO-VERTICAL DIAMETER

**Figure 5.9** Well-applied forceps blade alongside the fetal head.

This moves the tips of the forceps to lie centrally within the pelvis, avoiding trauma to the vaginal walls during the short rotation. Keep the handles elevated and rotate gently to DOA between contractions (i.e. move the handles to '12 o'clock'). Finally, bring the handles down to the horizontal plane and recheck the position of the blades to ensure that there has been no slippage around the fetal head. You are now ready to apply traction.

## Traction

- **Traction**: traction should be timed with uterine contractions unless there is acute fetal compromise. Moderate traction using arm and shoulder force only will be adequate. For mid-cavity birth, and the initial part of a low cavity birth, the aim is to apply traction *along the long axis of the mid pelvis*. The pelvic curve of the forceps follows the direction of the birth canal and lies along the straight arm of the 'J' shaped pelvic curve at mid-pelvis (Figure 5.10).

- **Pajot's manoeuvre**: Pajot's manoeuvre is used to encourage initial descent of the fetal head along the straight arm of the pelvic curve, through the mid and low pelvic cavities, until the head is 'crowning'. The operator applies *horizontal* traction force with the dominant hand, using the handles or shoulders of the forceps. The other hand applies *vertical force downwards* over the shanks. These two vector forces must be balanced to produce a resultant vector force that encourages the head to descend along the appropriate path, passing under the symphysis pubis (Figure 5.10).

The forceps handles should be kept more or less horizontal during traction and descent, until the occiput is emerging under the pubic arch. *The most common mistake seen is when the forceps handles are dropped 30 to 40 degrees below*

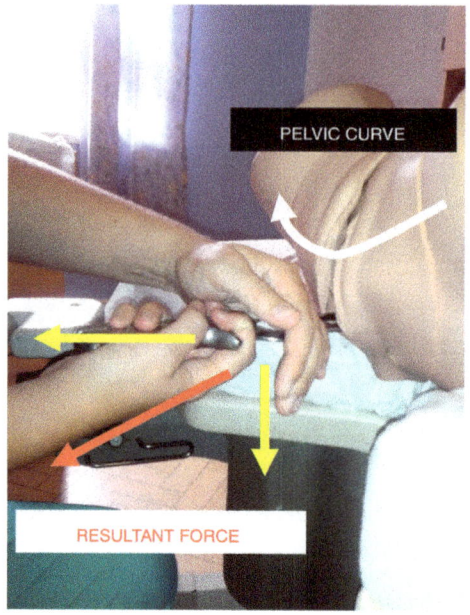

**Figure 5.10** The pelvic curve and force vectors associated with Pajot's manoeuvre.

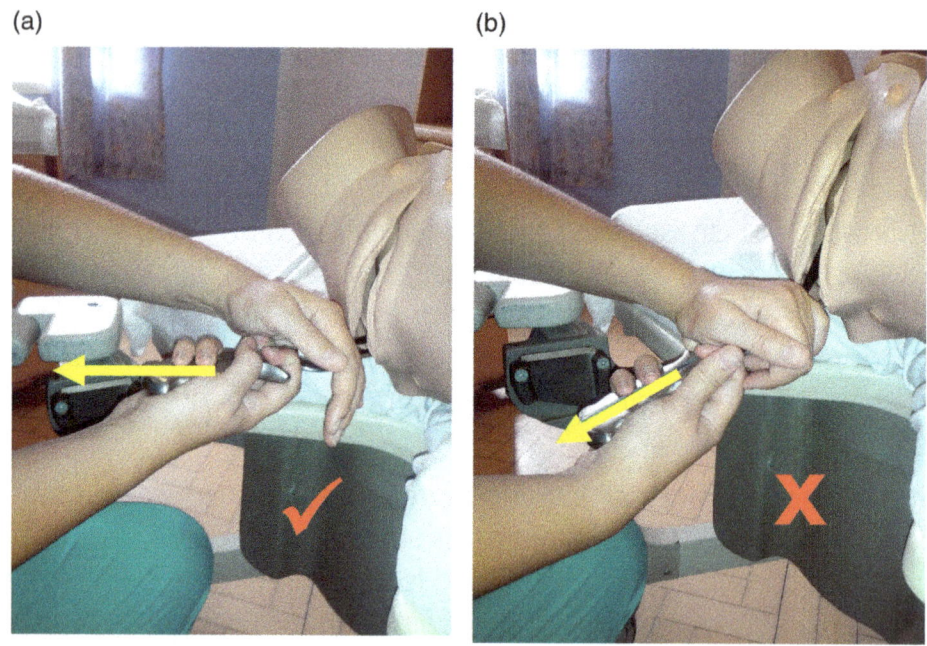

**Figure 5.11** Pajot's manoeuvre: correct and incorrect.

*the horizontal during initial traction* (Figure 5.11a and 5.11b). Dropping the handles results in the tips of the forceps moving anteriorly, which may damage the anterior vaginal wall (or bladder) when traction is applied.

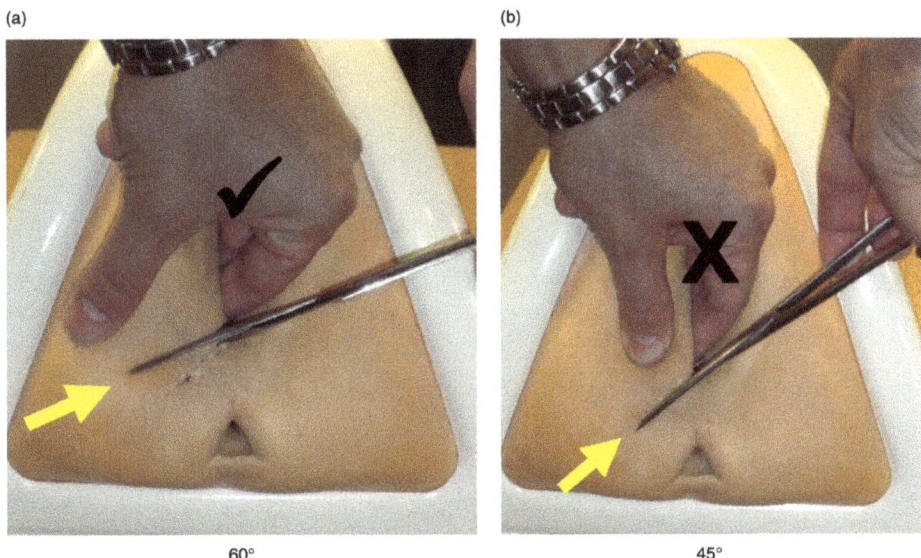

(a) 60°  (b) 45°

**Figure 5.12** Appropriate angle for episiotomy.

The fetal head will gradually descend until the occiput lies under the symphysis pubis. At that point the operator should stop using Pajot's manoeuvre. As the fetal head reaches the pelvic outlet/introitus, the perineum will distend and the need for an episiotomy can be assessed.

- **Episiotomy**: forceps births are associated with an increased risk of obstetric anal sphincter injury (OASI – 8–12%).[12] Mediolateral episiotomy directed laterally at an angle of at least 60 degrees in the direction of ischial tuberosity results in a lower incidence of anal sphincter tearing, anal incontinence and perineal pain (Figure 5.12).[1,16] RCOG guidance suggests that in the absence of robust evidence to support either routine or restrictive use of episiotomy at assisted vaginal birth, the decision should be tailored to the circumstances at the time and the preferences of the woman.[1] However, there is stronger evidence to support use of mediolateral episiotomy to prevent OASI at AVB for nulliparous women and for births using forceps.

- **Completing delivery of the head**: as the occiput emerges under the symphysis pubis (SP), it is important to minimise the risks of severe perineal trauma by using the following techniques:
  - ☐ *Stop using Pajot's manoeuvre,* as delivery of the head will now be completed by extension.
  - ☐ Ask the woman to stop active pushing in order to avoid rapid delivery of the head through the perineum.

(a)  (b)

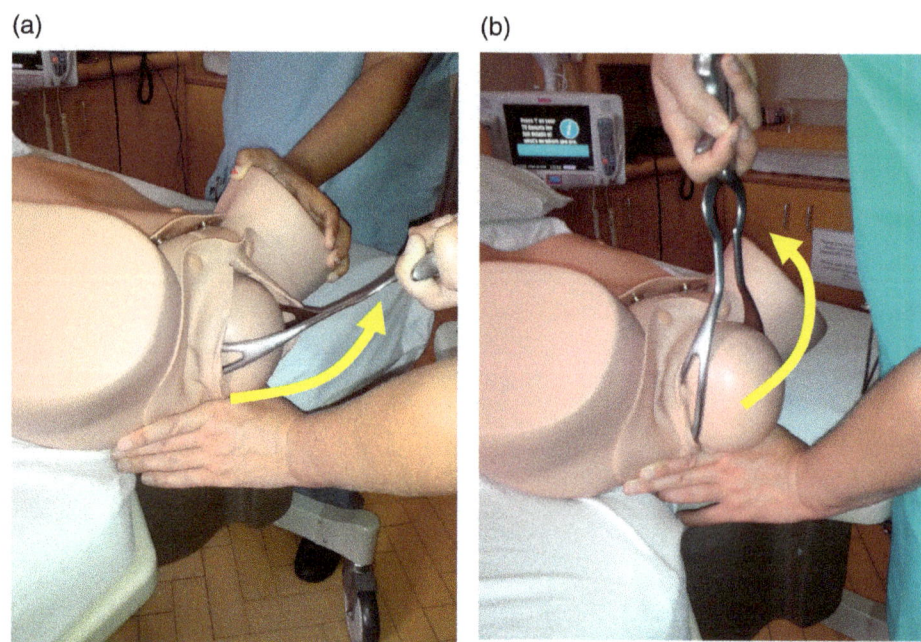

**Figure 5.13** Completing delivery of the head.

☐ In the absence of acute fetal compromise, aim for a slow delivery; the longer the perineal tissue is allowed to distend, the less likely severe perineal trauma will occur.

☐ As soon as the occiput emerges under the SP, start to raise the handles of the forceps in a gentle curve using one hand (Figure 5.13a), whilst the other hand guards the perineum using 'manual perineal protection' (MPP).

☐ MPP requires the accoucheur (or an assistant) to apply firm pressure to the central perineum with the curled up 3rd, 4th and 5th fingers, while the thumb and index finger are spread widely across the perineum. Drawing the thumb and index finger towards them midline reduces stretching forces in the perineal tissue.

☐ Timely and selective use of episiotomy is vital, and its use should be individualised, dependent on the clinical situation.

By the time the head is completely delivered, the forceps handles will be vertical over the SP (Figure 5.13b).

■ **Removing the forceps**: the forceps blades should be 'unlocked' and each blade should be removed separately: carefully slide each blade off around the head in the same way in which it was applied (Figure 5.14a–d).

■ **Completing the birth**: this mirrors the process of normal birth. Be aware of the increased risk of shoulder dystocia. Ask the mother if she would like the baby placed on her abdomen. Delayed cord clamping should be followed in

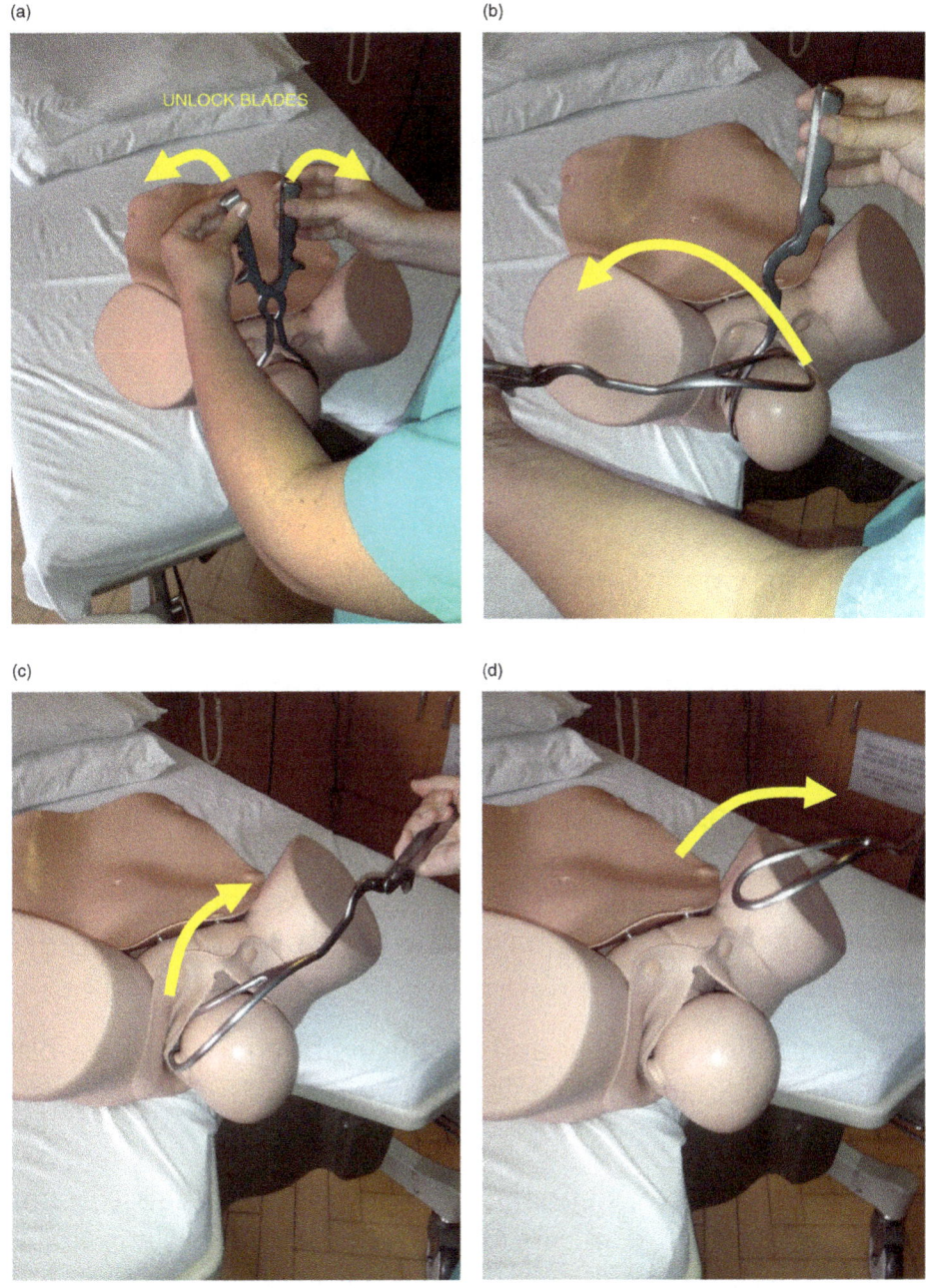

**Figure 5.14** Unlocking and removing the forceps.

the majority of cases and the third stage should be actively managed. Ensure that the placenta is complete.

- **Assessing for trauma post-birth**: the genital tract should be inspected systematically to detect trauma and prompt repair undertaken.

- **Antibiotic prophylaxis**: the 'ANODE' trial (n = 3,427) confirmed that routine use of single dose IV antibiotic prophylaxis following AVB (amoxicillin with clavulanic acid) significantly reduced confirmed or suspected postnatal infection compared to placebo (180 [11%] of 1,619 versus 306 [19%] of 1,606; RR 0·58, 95% CI 0·49–0·69; p < 0·0001).[17] This is now part of standard clinical practice in the UK.[1]

■ **Bladder care**: consider the need to insert an indwelling catheter. When regional analgesia has been used for a trial of AVB in theatre, an indwelling catheter should be inserted after the birth to prevent covert urinary retention, to be removed according to the local protocol.[1]

# Documentation and Debriefing the Patient

After every AVB the operator must ensure that a comprehensive, accurate and contemporaneous record is made, which is signed and dated appropriately.

This will include details of prior assessment, consent, the procedure itself and the initial condition of the baby (including Apgar scores, cord pH, need for resuscitation, etc. as per local protocols). Specific detail on the number of pulls, number of contractions, traction force *used*, etc. should be noted. Completion of the third stage of labour, assessment for trauma and consequent repair, swab and instrument count and estimated blood loss should also be recorded. Electronic records for AVB can enhance the amount of detail recorded for future reference.

The record should also give clear and specific instructions for post-birth care, including bladder drainage, analgesic requirements, VTE prophylaxis, perineal care, etc.

Follow-up of the mother for debriefing can be difficult because of early discharge policies and out-of-hours rota systems. However, it is vital that the operator aims to visit the mother before discharge home for a short, focused debrief. This will allow discussion about any questions or concerns that the mother may have. Women should be reassured that the risk of a forceps delivery in future pregnancies is usually very low.[1] All obstetricians should consider using a validated tool to assess patient perception of the AVB. The SaFE Patient Perception Score (PPS) is simple for patients to complete with high internal reliability.[18] Direct patient assessment of clinical practice can facilitate learning and appraisal. Low scores are infrequent but can be used to address concerns for individual operators. Women tend to highlight concerns about 'non-technical' rather than 'technical skills', which include matters related to decision-making, communication, etc. (see Chapter 3).

# Manual Rotation

An alternative to vacuum or Kielland's rotation is manual rotation from OT or OP positions. After successful manual rotation (MR), birth may be spontaneous or assisted (usually using forceps). MR is the most common technique used in the UK to correct malposition.[19,20] There is evidence that manual/digital rotation from a posterior to anterior position may reduce the number of AVBs[21,22] and caesarean sections.[22]

The techniques described vary. Digital rotation involves encouraging rotation of the head from the transverse towards an OA position by applying pressure on the lambdoidal or coronal suture of the fetal head during a contraction, aided by maternal effort. The aim is to encourage rotation, and this may result in spontaneous birth or an AVB.[19]

Manual rotation for persistent OP position involves placing the whole of the operator's hand within the vagina to lie in the lower pelvis behind the fetal head.[19] The hand acts as a 'surrogate' for the gutter formed by the pelvic floor muscles. For a left OP position, the right hand is inserted (vice versa for a right OP position). This requires gentle insertion, and adequate analgesia should be in place. For a multiparous woman, use of inhaled nitrous oxide ('Entonox') may be useful, but pudendal or regional blockade will usually be required for nulliparous women. The thumb is then positioned alongside the anterior fontanelle (Figure 5.15). The mother is asked to push with a contraction and the operator applies pressure with the thumb to flex the head. As flexion occurs, the head will start to rotate towards an OA position with minimal effort from the operator. When rotation has been achieved, the mother can be asked to push, aiming to complete the birth herself. If descent does not occur (or if

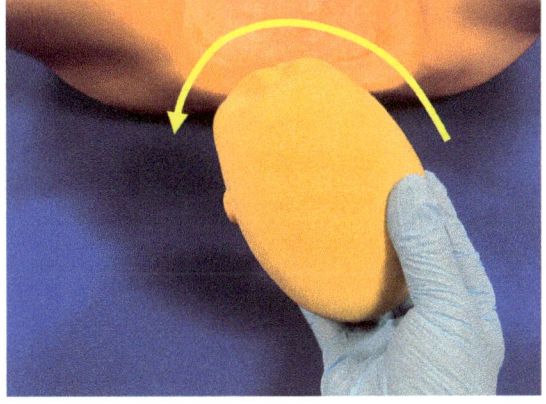

**Figure 5.15** Manual rotation.

the fetal condition requires intervention), the operator can proceed to complete delivery with forceps or vacuum.

(Note: the fetal head should not be disimpacted when using this technique for manual rotation.)

MR may be used *prophylactically* (pMR) at the start of the second stage to correct OP/OT position before pushing or *therapeutically* (tMR) to avoid instrumental rotation and delivery when the position remains OT or OP after pushing.[19] A small RCT of nulliparous women (n = 254) randomised to prophylactic MR or 'sham' MR did not confirm a reduction in the rate of assisted delivery.[23] The latest systematic review (n = 1,402; 7 studies) was a combination of both prophylactic and therapeutic interventions, and overall this suggests that MR is associated with a higher rate of spontaneous vaginal delivery: 64.9% versus 59.5% (RR = 1.09; 95% CI 1.03 to1.16; p = 0.005). However, the trials lacked the power to demonstrate an association between manual rotation and reductions in these consequences of OP, such as PPH or OASI. Neonatal outcomes did not differ between the groups.[24] Larger RCTs are required. The ROTATE trial commenced in the UK in 2022 and is a multicentre trial of 5,200 women from approximately 40 sites, who will be randomised to either: (1) therapeutic manual rotation (tMR) or (2) vacuum/Kielland's forceps rotation (the latter intervention is based on the skill set of the accoucheur). The trial will allow detection of a reduction in perineal trauma from 6% to 4% with 90% power.[25]

# Special Circumstances

## Traction and Birth in Low OP Position

If the head remains in a DOP position and is low cavity (i.e. 2 cm or more below the ischial spines), the option of non-rotational forceps can be considered (i.e. resulting in delivery in the 'face to pubes' position). *However, it is important to note that completing the birth in this position requires downwards traction to be maintained for longer and a large episiotomy is usually required.* The deflexed occiput predisposes to an increased risk of third- or fourth-degree tear. In this circumstance, there may be advantages to undertaking a vacuum-assisted birth, as rotation to OA position can occur even on the perineum. Mid-cavity OP positions may be rotated using vacuum, Kielland's or manual rotation.

## Face Presentation

Non-rotational forceps may be used when there is a need to expedite birth in the second stage in the presence of delay or fetal compromise. Face presentation is an absolute contra-indication to vacuum delivery but remember that non-rotational forceps may only be applied to a face presentation in the mento-anterior position. The forceps technique is similar to that outlined above for OP birth.

## Abandoning a Procedure and Use of Sequential Instruments

In undertaking a forceps birth, the operator must ensure that adequate progress is being made throughout the assisted birth process. Maintaining a 'willingness to abandon' the procedure is vital to ensure the safety of both the mother and the neonate. In particular, the operator must avoid using increased traction force or too many pulls when there is failure of descent. At times, the first instrument may fail and the situation should be critically reviewed before a second instrument is applied. Vacuum-assisted birth has a higher failure rate than forceps, and the second instrument used in most sequential attempts at vaginal birth is forceps.[26]

The decision to abandon the procedure after use of one instrument has to be balanced with the risks of a full dilatation caesarean section with increased maternal and neonatal morbidity.[1,27] There is clearly a difference between completing the birth using a second instrument *from the level of the pelvic outlet* and the use of a second instrument *following a failed attempt at mid-cavity rotation*. One example to consider would be a vacuum undertaken for delay associated with a transverse position just below the ischial spines. If there has been good descent and rotation, but the vacuum cup 'pops off' on or near the perineum, it would be reasonable to complete the birth using low cavity, non-rotational forceps (after carefully reassessment of position, etc.). A cohort study of nulliparous women concluded that the use of sequential instruments was associated with greater maternal and neonatal morbidity compared with forceps alone (anal sphincter tear = OR 1.8, 95% CI 1.1–2.9; umbilical artery pH < 7.10 = OR 3.0, 95% CI 1.7–5.5).[27] However, the majority of cases where use of a second instrument is planned should be discussed with a consultant before proceeding.

Updated RCOG guidance (2020) has made the following recommendations in terms of difficulties encountered during forceps delivery:[1]

■ Discontinue attempted forceps birth where the forceps cannot be applied easily, the handles do not approximate ('lock') easily or if there is a lack of progressive descent with moderate traction.

■ Discontinue attempted forceps birth if birth is not imminent following three pulls of a correctly applied instrument by an experienced operator.

■ If there is minimal descent with the first one or two pulls of the forceps, the operator should consider whether the application is suboptimal, the position has been incorrectly diagnosed or there is cephalopelvic disproportion. Less experienced operators should stop and seek a second opinion. Experienced operators should re-evaluate the clinical findings and either change approach or discontinue the procedure.

In terms of neonatal outcome:

■ Obstetricians should be aware of the potential neonatal morbidity following a failed attempt at forceps birth and should inform the neonatologist when this occurs to ensure appropriate management of the baby.

In terms of the need to proceed to an emergency second stage caesarean section:

■ Obstetricians should be aware of the increased risk of fetal head impaction at caesarean birth following a failed attempt at birth via forceps and should be prepared to disimpact the fetal head using recognised manoeuvres.

## Consultant Presence and Supervision

Forceps birth requires competence and confidence, both of which are acquired by practical experience. With reduced training time, trainees may be reluctant to attempt what they perceive as difficult procedures if the consultant is not on the labour ward.[28] Assisted vaginal birth should be performed by, or in the presence of, an operator who has the knowledge, skills and experience necessary to assess the woman, complete the procedure and manage any complications that arise, and the RCOG encourages trainees to ensure consultant presence is sought earlier if any concerns arise.[1]

Murphy et al. concluded that senior operators were less likely to proceed to caesarean section and there was less likelihood of major haemorrhage (OR 0.5, 95% CI 0.3–0.9).[29] In a small observational study (n = 32), Oláh confirmed that when a trainee decision to proceed directly to caesarean section in the second stage was followed by a consultant examination within 15 minutes, the decision was reversed, and successful assisted vaginal birth achieved in 63% of cases.[30] Another small cohort study (n = 50) confirmed that consultant presence for 'trials in theatre' significantly increased vaginal birth rates (70% [7/10] versus 30% [12/40]; $P < 0.05$).[28] Direct consultant input in more complex forceps births is not only a patient safety issue, but is an invaluable training opportunity, allowing immediate feedback for the trainee and with the potential to improve clinical technique.

## Trial of AVB in Theatre

RCOG guidance confirms that non-rotational low pelvic and lift out assisted vaginal births have a low probability of failure and most procedures can be conducted safely in a birth room.[1] AVBs that have a higher risk of failure should be considered a 'trial' and conducted in a place where immediate recourse to caesarean section can be undertaken. Factors that are associated with higher failure rates are maternal body mass index (BMI) >30, estimated fetal weight >4,000 g, OP position and mid-cavity birth, or when one-fifth of the head is palpable per abdomen. The incidence of trial of AVB in theatre is estimated at 2–5%. The most common reason for a 'trial in theatre' is to manage arrested progress in the second stage of labour at mid-cavity, which may be attributable to relative cephalopelvic disproportion, often associated with an OP position. Immediate resort to caesarean section is needed if the trial is unsuccessful. However, moving to theatre is associated with a longer decision to delivery interval (DDI) compared with AVB in the labour room (mean [SD] 30.0 [14.6] versus 14.5 [9.5] minutes) but is not associated with any increase in neonatal morbidity.[31] One problem associated with a trial in theatre is the potential loss of maternal assistance related to the 'density' of spinal/epidural blockade (often inserted in preparation for a possible caesarean section). This problem may be compounded by the use of vacuum techniques in theatre and consequently higher failure rates. The operator must individualise care and balance all aspects of safe delivery for both mother and baby. It is clear that not all rotational deliveries will require moving to the operating room environment, particularly when delivery is low cavity. The presence of potential fetal compromise requires critical assessment, balancing the potential delay associated with transfer to theatre with the potential to require urgent caesarean section if the trial is unsuccessful.

# The Role of Simulation in Training

RCOG guidance emphasises the importance of simulation training:

- Ensure obstetric trainees receive appropriate training in vacuum and forceps birth, including theoretical knowledge, simulation training and clinical training under direct supervision.

Simulation training in obstetrics not only allows the practice of assisted delivery techniques in a safe environment, but also improves the performance of individuals and obstetric teams. High-quality evidence confirms that simulated practice leads to improvement for obstetricians in both their technical and their communication skills.[32,33] Historically, practical obstetric skills were learned by observing an experienced colleague, followed by gaining further experience by supervision and observed practice directly on patients. Patient safety has been another driver for increased use of simulation in training for forceps birth. Use of pelvic mannequins is not new and was actively promoted in the eighteenth century by the French midwife Madame du Coudray. Simple mannequins allow the trainee to develop both technical skills and a systematic approach to forceps birth. They build confidence, with trainers able to objectively assess trainees' progress. There are an increasing number of more sophisticated simulators: Dupuis et al. have developed a spatial tracking system that assesses the trajectory of the forceps blade tip during insertion, used with a childbirth simulator.[34] Objective assessment of traction force during simulation training for shoulder dystocia demonstrated a significant reduction in applied traction force after training.[35] Subsequent studies confirmed a reduction in brachial plexus injury in hospitals that had undertaken the training programme.

Mannequin training in non-rotational forceps should focus on the three main aspects of technical skill that need to be mastered, namely: careful assessment and forceps application, appropriate traction skills and active perineal protection. Other elements of simulation training concentrate on the equally important area of 'non-technical skills', which are highly relevant to undertaking a safe forceps birth (i.e. situational awareness, decision-making, task management, team working, communication).[36] Simulation is an adjunct to clinical exposure but is an important step in ensuring better training in the use of forceps. The RCOG supplies other online video learning resources for forceps skills.[37]

# Summary

Non-rotational forceps delivery and manual rotation remain important components of the skill set that the obstetrician should be able to offer women in contemporary obstetric practice. A skilled practitioner must be aware of the correct clinical situation in which forceps can ensure maximum benefit to mother and baby. Rotational delivery skills must be maintained, balanced by an appropriate rate for second stage caesarean section. Manual rotation is a skill that practitioners should learn, and may be of particular benefit to multiparous women with a malposition. The roles of prophylactic and therapeutic manual rotation require assessment within large, high-quality research trials. Simulation has a vital role in developing assisted birth skills and must include training in both 'technical' and 'non-technical' skills.

# References

1.  Murphy DJ, Strachan BK, Bahl R, on behalf of the Royal College of Obstetricians Gynaecologists. Assisted Vaginal Birth (Greentop Guideline No 26). *BJOG* 2020; 127(9): e70-e112. doi.org/10.1111/1471–0528.16092

2.  NHS Digital. NHS Maternity Statistics, England 2016–17. https://digital.nhs.uk/data-and-information/publications/statistical/nhs-maternity-statistics/2016-17

3.  Public Health Scotland. Births in Scottish Hospitals (year ending March 2021). Published online November 2021. Accessed 20 Sept 2022. www.publichealthscotland.scot/media/10489/2021-11-30-births-report.pdf

4.  Europeristat. European Perinatal Health Report 2015. Published online 26 November 2018. Accessed 20 Sept 2022. www.europeristat.com/index.php/reports/european-perinatal-health-report-2015.html

5.  Boucoiran I, Valerio L, Bafghi A, Delotte J, Bongain A. Spatula-assisted deliveries: a large cohort of 1065 cases. *Eur J Obstet Gynecol Reprod Biol*. 2010; 151(1):46–51.

6.  Verma GL, Spalding JJ, Wilkinson MD et al. Instruments for assisted vaginal birth. Cochrane Database of Systematic Reviews 2021, Issue 9. Art. No.: CD005455. https://doi.org/10.1002/14651858.CD005455.pub3

7.  Alexander JM, Leveno KJ, Rouse DJ et al. Comparison of maternal and infant outcomes from primary cesarean delivery during the second compared with first stage of labor. *Obstet Gynecol*. 2007; 109(4): 917–21.

8.  Yeo L, Romero R. Sonographic evaluation in the second stage of labour to improve the assessment of labor progress and its outcome. *Ultrasound Obstet Gynecol*. 2009; 33(3):253–8.

9.  Ramphul M, Kennelly M, Murphy DJ. Establishing the accuracy and acceptability of abdominal ultrasound to define the foetal head position in the second stage of labour: a validation study. *Eur J Obstet Gynecol Reprod Biol*. 2012; 164:35–39.

10. Royal College of Obstetricians and Gynaecologists. Information for you – assisted vaginal birth (ventouse or forceps). RCOG, London, April 2020. Accessed Sept 2022. www.rcog.org.uk/media/2p4fh2kd/pi-vaginal-birth-final-28042020.pdf

11. Chan SW, Tulloch E, Cooper ES et al. Montgomery and informed consent: where are we now? BMJ 2017; 357:j2224.

12. Royal College of Obstetrics and Gynaecologists. Operative vaginal delivery: consent Advice No.11. July 2010; London: RCOG. Accessed 20 Sept 2022. www.rcog.org.uk/guidance/browse-all-guidance/consent-advice/operative-vaginal-delivery-consent-advice-no-11/

13. Royal College of Obstetricians and Gynaecologists. Obtaining valid consent. Clinical Governance Advice No. 6. London: RCOG; 2008. Accessed 20 September 2022. www.rcog.org.uk/guidance/browse-all-guidance/clinical-governance-advice/obtaining-valid-consent-clinical-governance-advice-no-6/

14. Bolton H. The perils of taking written consent for operative delivery during labour. BJOG 2015; 122(9): 1251. https://doi.org/10.1111/1471-0528.13496

15. Bahl R, Murphy DJ, Strachan B. Qualitative analysis by interviews and video recordings to establish the components of a skilled low-cavity non-rotational vacuum delivery. *BJOG*. 2009; 116(2):319–26.

16. Kalis V, Landsmanova J, Bednarova B et al. Evaluation of the incision angle of mediolateral episiotomy at 60 degrees. *Int J Gynaecol Obstet*. 2011; 112(3):220–4.

17. Knight M, Chiocchia V, Partlett C et al. ANODE collaborative group. Prophylactic antibiotics in the prevention of infection after operative vaginal delivery (ANODE): a multicentre randomised controlled trial. *Lancet*. 2019; 393(10189):2395–2403. DOI: 10.1016/S0140-6736(19)30773-1

18. Siassakos D, Clark J, Sibanda T et al. A simple tool to measure patient perceptions of operative birth. *BJOG* 2009; DOI: 10.1111/j.1471-0528.2009.02363.x.

19. O' Brien S, Jordan S, Siassakos D. The role of manual rotation in avoiding and managing OVD. *Best Pract Res: Clin Obstet Gynaecol* 2019; 56: 69–80. https://doi.org/10.1016/j.bpobgyn.2018.12.001

20. UK-ARCOG, Tempest N. ReDEFINe (Rotational DElivery at Full dIlatatioN): a national prospective service evaluation of deliveries complicated by malposition in the second stage. *BJOG* 2017; 124 (Supp 5): 28. Accessed 20 Sept 2022. http://ukarcog.org/wp-content/uploads/2018/01/ReDEFINe-facts-and-figures-poster.pdf

21. Vayssie C, Beucher G, Dupuis O et al. Instrumental delivery: clinical practice guidelines from the French College of Gynaecologists and Obstetricians. *Eur J Obstet Gynecol Reprod Biol.* 20111; 159:43–8.

22. Reichman O, Gdansky E, Latinsky B, Labi S, Samueloff A. Digital rotation from occipito-posterior to occipito-anterior decreases the need for caesarean section. *Eur J Obstet Gynecol Reprod Biol.* 2008; 136:25–8.

23. Bertholdt C, Morel O, Zuily S, Ambroise-Grandjean G. Manual rotation of occiput posterior or transverse positions: a systematic review and meta-analysis of randomized controlled trials. *Am J Obstet Gynecol.* 2022 ; 226(6):781–93. doi: https://doi.org/10.1016/j.ajog.2021.11.033 Epub 2021 Nov 17. PMID: 34800396.

24. Phipps H, Hyett JA, Kuah S et al. Persistent occiput posterior position outcomes following manual rotation: a randomized controlled trial. *Am J Obstet Gynecol MFM.* 2021 ;3(2):100306. doi: https://doi.org/10.1016/j.ajogmf.2021.100306 Epub 2021 Jan 6. PMID: 33418103.

# Chapter 6
# Rotational Forceps

Karl SJ Oláh

---

## Key Learning Points

- Kielland's forceps have been shown to be associated with a high success rate in terms of birth in cases of fetal malposition.

- Rotational forceps are an instrument that every labour ward specialist should endeavour to become experienced with.

- Know, do not guess, the fetal position and station prior to any assisted birth.

- Choose the instrument for birth most appropriate for the circumstances – be familiar with all instruments, not just one.

- Rotational forceps should be conducted in theatre, usually under spinal or epidural anaesthesia.

- The use of rotational forceps requires a tactile sensory input through the instrument; they are not to be used with force.

- The angle of traction must follow the angle of the birth canal, which, in view of the lack of pelvic curve on the instrument, is more acute (a more downward pull towards the floor) than that used with traction forceps.

- Do not force any stage of the procedure (application of blades, rotation). Do not be afraid to abandon the procedure and perform a caesarean section.

- Manual rotation and ventouse are alternatives to the use of Kielland's forceps.

---

In 1915, Christian Kielland (1871–1941) first described his forceps to achieve birth from the mid-pelvis in cases of malrotation (OP and OT positions of the fetal head).[1,2] Kielland (sometimes spelt Kjelland) described his forceps to be applied for a condition that would not be applicable today (the fetal head arrested in a high transverse or OP position), and in a manner which would be considered dangerous in modern practice. However, the instrument was adopted and adapted in the twentieth century and became popular for use by obstetricians in cases of malposition.

Most of the studies of Kielland's forceps, albeit with some exceptions,[3] do not show any significant excess of fetal or maternal complications as a result of their use.[4–7] Concern arose in the 1980s when there were a few high-profile medico-legal cases, and there was a lot of optimism that the ventouse could do the same job but with fewer adverse effects.[8] More recently, Kielland's forceps have been shown to be associated, in the hands of (or under the supervision of) experienced accoucheurs, with a high success rate in terms of birth (failure to effect birth is approximately 10% in most series) and a low maternal and neonatal morbidity.[7,9–12]

Indeed, the suggestion to consign the instrument to the obstetric museum was first made in the 1980s, and the final death knell was sounded by the studies comparing it unfavourably with the ventouse.[13] A recognised disadvantage of the ventouse is its higher rate of failure to achieve a vaginal birth compared with forceps.[14] One study has shown similarities in the rate of levator ani muscle injury or avulsion for forceps delivery when compared to the ventouse.[15] The multicentre ROTATE RCT will provide robust evidence with regard to the impact of rotational methods on the pelvic floor (https://fundin gawards.nihr.ac.uk/award/NIHR127818).

In the meantime, recent data support the continued use of this instrument in selected cases if there is an experienced senior obstetrician to conduct or supervise.

A rising trend amongst clinicians preferring manual rotation has also been observed. This may be a result of the perceived need to rotate a baby to achieve delivery, but a reluctance to employ an instrument with a poor anecdotal perception, and they have not been instructed in their use. Manual rotation is a viable alternative to Kielland's forceps and has been shown to be similarly effective in some studies. One study has shown that there are more cases of shoulder dystocia in the Kielland's group,[7] perhaps suggesting that they may be more effective where there is true disproportion between maternal and fetal diameter (and possible asynclitism – not formally corrected in manual rotation). However, this study was conducted in a single centre contemporaneously with a global effort to recognise shoulder dystocia – this may have increased the rate of diagnosis of shoulder dystocia without any change in the underlying mechanism of birth between rotational forceps and manual rotation. There has been recent concern about the increasing number of caesarean sections that are being performed in the second stage of labour, and some evidence that this may be, at least in part, due to a 'deskilling' in the art of operative vaginal birth, in particular the knowledge and use of forceps.[16–21]

Second stage caesarean section is perhaps one of the most challenging operative deliveries that we can be faced with, and guidelines in most centres would advise the presence of a 'senior obstetrician', in most cases a consultant, for such deliveries.[22] A deeply engaged head and the distortion of the anatomy can lead to significant trauma to the mother, and to the fetus. Second stage caesarean section is associated with long-term sequelae, in addition to the obvious vaginal and uterine trauma, including a significantly increased risk of preterm birth and abnormally invasive placenta in subsequent pregnancies.[22–25]

Recent attempts at reducing caesarean section rates have highlighted a need for further training in operative vaginal birth,[16,21] including all tools useful for undertaking successful operative vaginal births.

# Malposition

## Transverse Position and Transverse Arrest

True 'deep transverse arrest', which is associated with CPD, is rare. Most cases in which the fetus is found to be in a transverse position are attributable to some degree of deflexion and a failure of the fetal head to rotate, generally as a result of an epidural block that has altered the muscular component of the rotational mechanism.[26] Kielland's original application of the forceps to a fetus in a transverse position was probably because they were applied to a high head that had not yet had a chance to undergo rotation in the mid-pelvis. True transverse arrest will be associated with caput, moulding and asynclitism.

## Asynclitism

Asynclitism is the oblique presentation of the fetal head in labour, and it is important in the context of Kielland's forceps as it is corrected by the sliding lock on the instrument. Asynclitism may result from dystocia rather than being the cause of it and a comprehensive understanding of the process is required. As a result of asynclitism in a transverse arrest, either the anterior or the posterior parietal bone presents.

In anterior parietal presentation (Naegele's obliquity), the posteriorly lying parietal bone is arrested by the promontory of the sacrum causing the anterior parietal bone to be that presenting to the examining fingers (Figure 6.1). In the posterior parietal bone presentation (Litzmann's obliquity), the anterior parietal bone is arrested at the symphysis while the posterior parietal bone engages in the brim (Figure 6.2). This latter situation is often considered less favourable than the former and is also a much rarer presentation.[27]

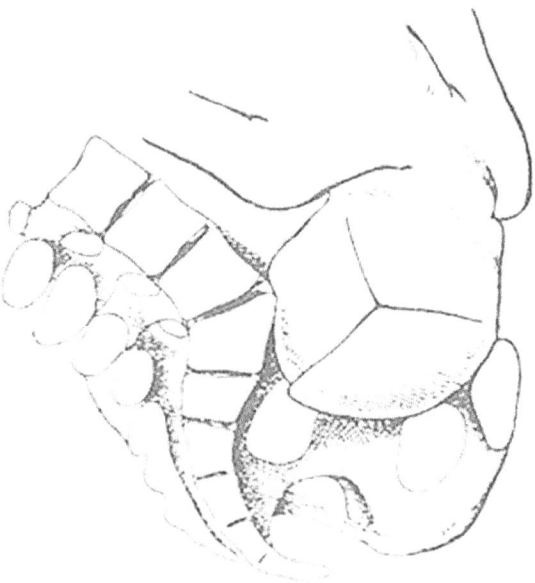

**Figure 6.1** Anterior parietal presentation (Naegele's obliquity).

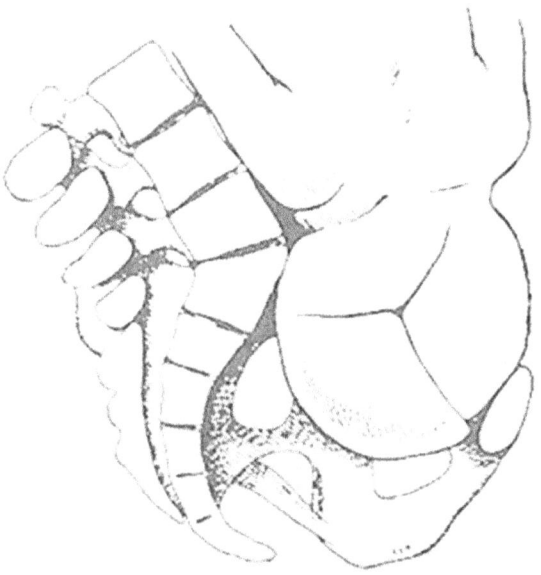

**Figure 6.2** Posterior parietal presentation (Litzmann's obliquity).

## Occipito-posterior Position

The appropriate management of the baby in an OP position remains one of the major challenges to the modern obstetrician. When birth is delayed in the second stage, delivery is usually possible with either Kielland's forceps or ventouse[12,28] but training to use each tool competently is equally important as the choice of tool. Using traction forceps to bring the baby out 'face to pubes' is more likely to result in trauma and increases fetal and maternal morbidity. It has been recognised for many years that where the baby is bought out 'face to pubes' the amount of trauma to the mother and baby is often excessive, with an increased incidence of third- and fourth-degree tears. The dimensions at the pelvic outlet required for birth in an OP position are greater as the fetal head cannot flex and then extend around the symphysis as it does in an occipito-anterior (OA) position.

# Kielland's Forceps – An Instrument for Modern Obstetric Practice

The modern obstetrician should be able to assess a clinical situation and then decide which instrument is best suited to effect a safe birth. Rotational forceps, rotational vacuum extraction and manual rotation have a place for those deliveries that require definitive rotation. They should be considered an excellent instrument in OP position of the fetal head in the hands of competent and trained accoucheurs,[7,9,29,30] and may be a useful tool where there is a transverse position and a suspicion of true deep transverse arrest. Essentially, a good practitioner should have access to and experience of all these instruments. Inability to use Kielland's forceps deprives the accoucheur of a tool par excellence for birth of a baby in an OP position.

## General Features of the Forceps

The measurements of the forceps are not important. However, the features of the instrument (Figure 6.3) that are important are:

- The sliding lock. This makes the instrument unique in its ability to correct asynclitism associated with obstructed labour.
- The absence of any appreciable pelvic curve. This means that when the forceps are rotated about their axis, the ends of the blades do not describe a circle, they rotate around their axis. Trying the same thing with Simpson's or Neville Barnes forceps results in a large circular motion of the forceps tips.
- The direction indicator markers. These are small nodular metal markings on the shanks or handles that indicate which way the occiput should be in relation to the forceps.

The forceps themselves are light, with fenestrated blades and with handles that, if compressed, will approximate the blades.

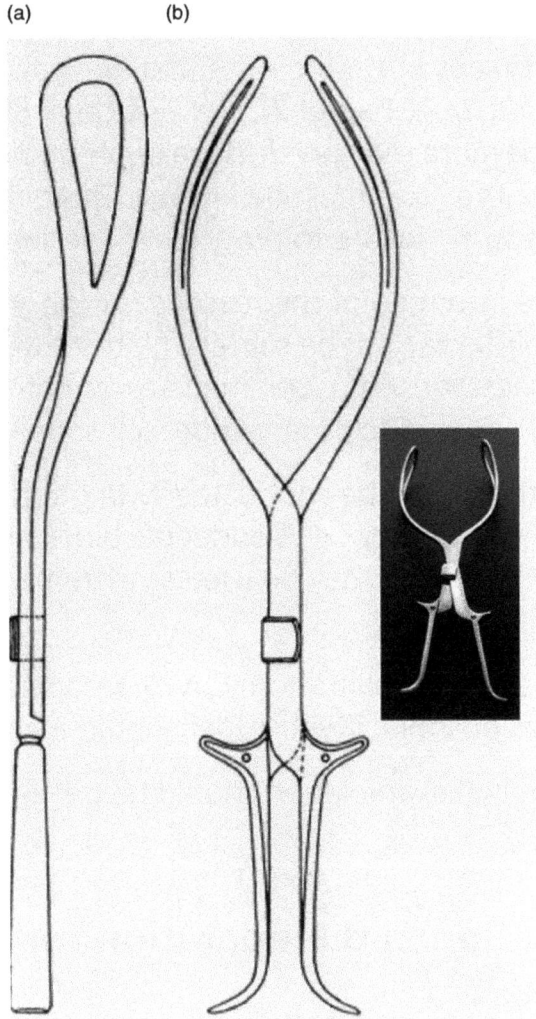

**Figure 6.3** Kielland's rotational forceps. Note the sliding lock (a) and the lack of a pelvic curve (b). The blades are fenestrated to reduce the weight of the instrument.

## Who Should Be Using Kielland's Forceps?

It is essential that Kielland's forceps are used only by obstetricians with the necessary training and experience. Unlike the ventouse, which unfortunately is sometimes used without the position of the fetal head being known with certainty, with Kielland's forceps the position of the fetal head must be known precisely. In addition, because the Kielland's forceps require experience and some degree of sensitivity and feedback through the instrument with regard to tissue resistance, it is expected that use of the Kielland's forceps would take place only once a practitioner is confident with traction forceps, and has had training, experience and confirmed and externally validated competence in the use of rotational forceps.

## Prerequisites and Contra-Indications

For a safe Kielland's forceps birth, the rules that apply to any assisted vaginal birth should be followed (see Chapter 2).[22,27] The cervix should be fully dilated. The head should not be more than one fifth palpable above the pelvic brim. The position and station of the head must be known. There must be a valid reason to perform the AVB (usually failure to progress in the second stage of labour).

The woman should be informed of the reasons for the AVB and, if there is a possibility that the birth may not be successful, the consent for such must be obtained.[22,31] The anaesthetist must be made aware of the possibility of a caesarean birth and a multidisciplinary approach should always be followed.

Kielland's forceps births should be conducted with good analgesia – usually a spinal or topped-up epidural block. A pudendal block alone will probably not be adequate for most cases but may be used in extremis. Delivery should usually be attempted in theatre.

The woman should be placed in lithotomy. A clean operative field should be established as much as possible. The bladder should always be emptied.

Finally, a thorough vaginal examination should be performed to establish the findings.

## Vaginal Examination and Preparation for Application of Forceps

It may seem de rigeur to perform a vaginal examination before an AVB. However, it has been reported that the findings of vaginal examinations performed by trainees suggest either a lack of avidity in establishing the fetal position, or a bias in the vaginal assessment findings to try to avoid an AVB in favour of a caesarean section.[18] When performing a vaginal examination before a Kielland's forceps birth, it is important to try to get it right.

Always document all the features of the vaginal findings, including the dilatation, the fetal station, the degree of moulding, caput and any other features that may be relevant, such as prominence of the ischial spines or narrowness of the subpubic arch. Also note whether there is a lot of space around the fetal head in the pelvis. Note any asynclitism and try and establish whether it is an anterior or posterior parietal bone presentation. Finally, and most importantly, the position needs to be established. Using the occiput as the denominator, describe the position as LOT, LOP, direct OP, direct ROT or ROT.

If there is caput, feel for the fontanelles and suture lines. Remember that the backs of the parietal bones have a serrated surface. Also, where there is continuing doubt, feel for the ears of the fetus. Where there is marked deflexion make sure that you feel for a nose or eye sockets in case it is a brow presentation.

Some obstetricians prefer to check the fetal position by ultrasound.[32] While this may be a useful and more accurate way to check the fetal position, it in no way should replace the vaginal examination. Additionally, there is no published evidence that yet demonstrates an improvement in either maternal or neonatal outcomes following the use of ultrasound determination of fetal position over manual examination only. Those that prefer the use of ultrasound should make a full assessment digitally first and then check their findings ultrasonically if they desire. There is so much more that can be gleaned from a digital examination than from ultrasonic imaging alone. For example, the degree of moulding, the station, and an assessment of the capacity of the pelvis are all aspects that an experienced obstetrician will consider.

Once the position is identified, and you are happy that a Kielland's forceps birth is the most appropriate birth in your hands, you are now ready to apply the forceps. Take the forceps and assemble them in front of the perineum. Remember that the small buttons on the shanks of the forceps indicate where the occiput should be. Therefore, assemble them with the small buttons pointing towards the occiput. Finally, lubricate the forceps with obstetric cream and prepare to apply the blades.

## Application

### General

The forceps should be held with a light grip, and not clenched with the intention of rotating the fetal head come what may. Parry-Jones,[33] in his book on the subject, suggested using the tips of the fingers, and there is much to commend this approach.

### Transverse Position

With a fetus in the transverse position there are two options for forceps application:

■ **Direct application**. The anterior blade is applied first. The blade is positioned with the direction indicator knob pointing towards the occiput, and the blade passed over the fetal head in a similar way to that which is used when applying traction forceps posteriorly (Figure 6.4). Once the

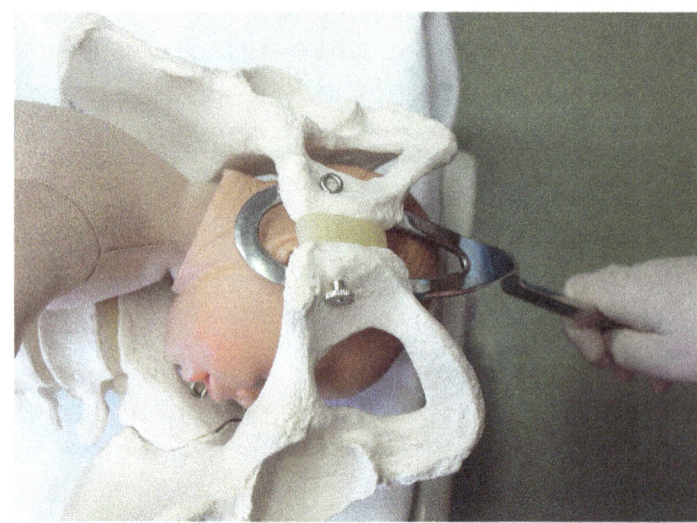

**Figure 6.4** Transverse position: direct application of the anterior blade.

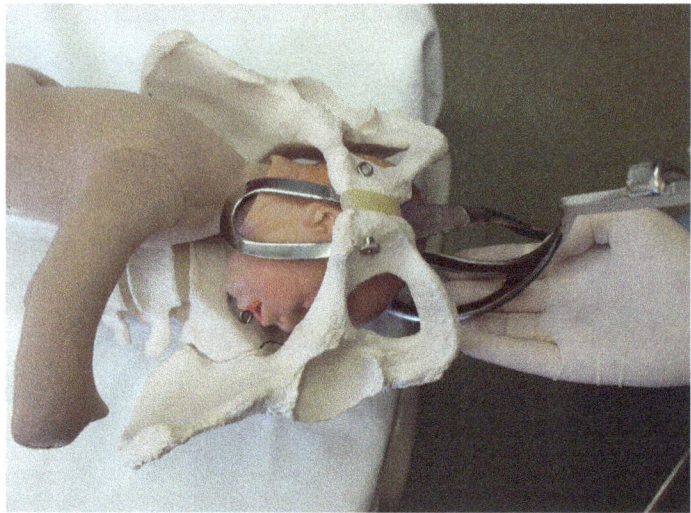

**Figure 6.5** Transverse position: direct application of the posterior blade. Once inserted, the blades are locked and asynclitism corrected.

anterior blade is positioned, the posterior blade is passed into the sacral hollow (Figure 6.5). The forceps blade should be slid in close to the head to prevent soft tissue injury. If there is difficulty in applying the posterior blade, often said to be due to the protrusion of the sacral promontory, the blade may be wandered slightly to the side, in front of the sacroiliac joint, then wandered back into the midline. The blades are approximated, asynclitism is corrected and rotation may be then attempted between contractions.

■ **Wandering application**. Where there is difficulty in applying the anterior blade, the anterior blade is first inserted posteriorly, and then wandered over the sinciput or the occiput (classically the sinciput). Once in position, the posterior blade is inserted. Again, asynclitism is corrected before attempting rotation.

### Occipito-posterior Position

Where the fetal position is OP, the forceps blades are applied directly, in a similar way to that used for traction forceps. The left blade is inserted first after assembling the forceps in front of the perineum and using the direction indicators on the forceps to have them facing the correct way.

On applying the right blade, the forceps are approximated and asynclitism corrected. Do not force the forceps in, and do not try to close the forceps against resistance. The higher the fetal head in the pelvis, the closer to vertical the forceps should be expected to be at the end of the application, a marked difference from the position of non-rotational forceps.

## Rotation

The first rule for rotation with Kielland's forceps is that it should not be forced. The second rule for rotation with Kielland's forceps is that it should not be forced. Rotation takes place usually after slight upwards displacement to disengage the head from the surrounding structures, and then rotation, which is conducted by 'feeling' the way around the pelvis, usually by the shortest route to obtain an anterior position. Of essence is that force is not applied – a gentle 'feel' so the head follows the line of least resistance is what is required. Once the head reaches the OA position, a characteristic 'clunk' is often felt through the forceps as the head fits into the pelvis.

## Traction

Traction on Kielland's forceps is in the direction of the birth canal. Because of the lack of a pelvic curve on the instrument, this means that traction will be more acutely angled towards the floor. Once the head has descended, traction must follow the angle of the canal around the symphysis pubis, and traction then will be more conventional, almost directly towards the operator, then slightly upwards as the head is delivered over the perineum.

As for the need for an episiotomy, this should be judged individually. Although not routine, one will be required on most occasions.

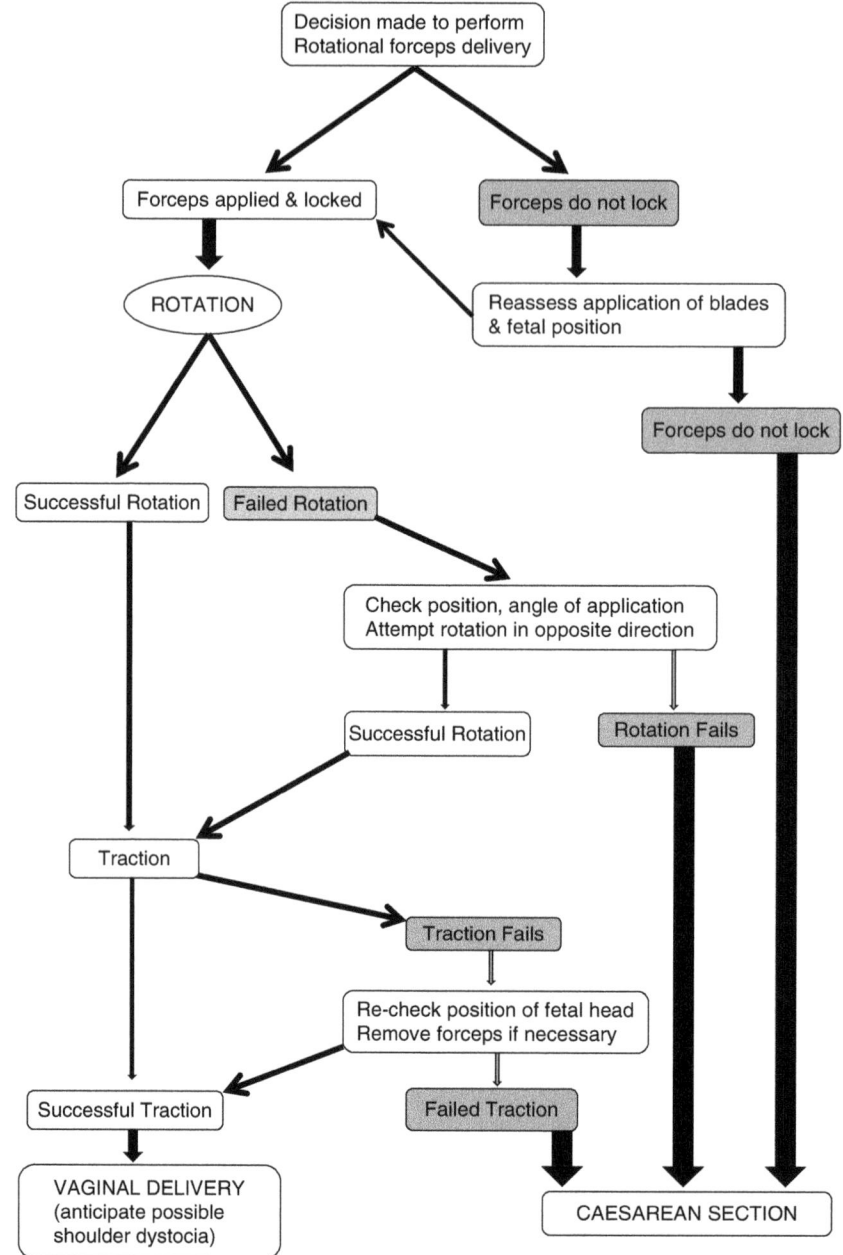

**Figure 6.6** Simplified algorithm for rotational forceps delivery: consent and debrief would be required at all stages. Also consider other rotational methods.

## Complications and How to Avoid Them

Any attempted AVB will occasionally result in maternal and neonatal adverse outcomes. Most are minor. To reduce the probability of severe adverse outcomes it is important to follow the rules closely and not to deviate from them. Do not force the blades in. Do not try to approximate the blades if they do not fit together properly. Do not force rotation.

Nerve injuries in the mother are possible but are usually transient. Fetal injury is also uncommon as long as the rules are followed. However, despite these minimal detrimental effects it is important to state that attempted rotational operative birth with Kielland's forceps is usually associated with fewer short- and long-term maternal and neonatal adverse outcomes than the alternative – a caesarean section in the second stage of labour.[9,25,34]

## Acknowledgements

Thanks to Olivia Oláh for her photographic expertise.

# References

1. Oláh KS. In praise of Kielland's forceps. Bjog Int J Obstetrics Gynaecol. 2002;109(5):492–4.

2. Kielland C. Über die Anlegung der Zange am nicht rotierten Kopf mit Beschreibung eines neuen Zangenmodelles und einer neuen Anlegungsmethode. Gynecol Obstet Inves. 1916;43(1):48–78.

3. Baker PN, Johnson IR. A study of the effect of rotational forceps delivery on fetal acid-base balance. Acta Obstet Gyn Scan. 1994;73(10):787–9.

4. Caughey AB, Sandberg PL, Zlatnik MG et al. Forceps compared with vacuum: rates of neonatal and maternal morbidity. Obstetrics Gynecol. 2006;107(3):740.

5. Johanson RB, Heycock E, Carter J et al. Maternal and child health after assisted vaginal delivery: five-year follow up of a randomised controlled study comparing forceps and ventouse. Bjog Int J Obstetrics Gynaecol. 2014;121 Suppl 7(s7):23–8.

6. Healy DL, Quinn MA, Pepperell RJ. Rotational delivery of the fetus: Kielland's forceps and two other methods compared. Bjog Int J Obstetrics Gynaecol. 1982;89(7):501–6.

7. O'Brien S, Day F, Lenguerrand E et al. Rotational forceps versus manual rotation and direct forceps: a retrospective cohort study. Eur J Obstet Gyn R B. 2017;212:119–25.

8. Herabutya Y, O-Prasertsawat P, Boonrangsimant P. Kielland's forceps or ventouse – a comparison. Bjog Int J Obstetrics Gynaecol. 1988;95(5):483–7.

9. Giacchino T, Karkia R, Zhang W et al. Kielland's rotational forceps delivery: a comparison of maternal and neonatal outcomes with rotational ventouse or second stage caesarean section deliveries. Eur J Obstet Gyn R B. 2020;254:175–80.

10. Tempest N, Hart A, Walkinshaw S, Hapangama DK. A re-evaluation of the role of rotational forceps: retrospective comparison of maternal and perinatal outcomes following different methods of birth for malposition in the second stage of labour. Bjog Int J Obstetrics Gynaecol [Internet]. 2013 ;120(10):1277–84. message:%3C20151214135111 .544944B82DB@nhs-pd1e-esg005.ad1.nhs.net%3E

11. Stock SJ, Josephs K, Farquharson S et al. Maternal and neonatal outcomes of successful Kielland's rotational forceps delivery. Obstetrics Gynecol. [Internet]. 2013;121(5):1032–9. message:%3C20151214135111.544944B82DB@nhs-pd1e-esg005.ad1.nhs.net%3E

12. Bahl R, Van deVenne M, Macleod M, Strachan B, Murphy DJ. Maternal and neonatal morbidity in relation to the instrument used for mid-cavity rotational operative vaginal delivery: a prospective cohort study. Bjog Int J Obstetrics Gynaecol. 2013;120(12):1526–33.

13. Burke N, Field K, Mujahid F, Morrison JJ. Use and safety of Kielland's forceps in current obstetric practice. Obstetrics Gynecol. 2012;120(4):766–70.

14. O'Mahony F, Hofmeyer GJ, Menon V. Choice of instruments for assisted vaginal delivery. O'Mahony F, editor. Cochrane Db Syst Rev. 2010;(11):CD005455.

15. García-Mejido JA, Fernández-Palacín A, Barby MJB et al. A comparable rate of levator ani muscle injury in operative vaginal delivery (forceps and vacuum) according to the characteristics of the instrumentation. Acta Obstet Gyn Scan. 2019;98(6):729–36.

16. Sinha P, Dutta A, Langford K. Instrumental delivery: how to meet the need for improvements in training. Obstetrician Gynaecol. 2010;12(4):265–71.

17. Unterscheider J, McMenamin M, Cullinane F. Rising rates of caesarean deliveries at full cervical dilatation: a concerning trend. *Eur J Obstet Gyn R B.* 2011;157(2):141–4.

18. Oláh KS. Reversal of the decision for caesarean section in the second stage of labour on the basis of consultant vaginal assessment. J Obstet Gynaecol [Internet]. 2005;25(2):115–6. message:%3C20160201144906.2B157449038@nhs-pd1e-esg006.ad1.nhs.net%3E

19. Lewis EA, Barr C, Thomas K. The mode of delivery in women taken to theatre at full dilatation: does consultant presence make a difference? J Obstet Gynaecol. 2011;31(3):229–31.

20. Chung W-H, Li Y-Y, Kong C-W, To WW-K. Association between rates of second-stage caesarean section and instrumental delivery. Hong Kong J Gynaecol Obstetrics Midwifery. 2019;19(2):89–95.

21. Tempest N, Lane S, Hapangama D ; UK Audit Research Trainee Collaborative in Obstetrics, Gynaecology (UK-ARCOG). Babies in occiput posterior position are significantly more likely to require an emergency cesarean birth compared with babies in occiput transverse position in the second stage of labor: a prospective observational study. Acta Obstet Gyn Scan. 2020;99(4):537–45.

22. Murphy DJ, Strachan BK, Bahl R on behalf of the Royal College of Obstetricians and Gynaecologists Assisted Vaginal Birth: Green-Top Guideline No. 26. Bjog Int J Obstetrics Gynaecol. 2020;127: e70–e112.

23. Watson HA, Carter J, David AL, Seed PT, Shennan AH. Full dilation cesarean section: a risk factor for recurrent second-trimester loss and preterm birth. Acta Obstetricia et Gynecologica Scandinavica. 2017;96(9):1100–5.

24. Bahl R, Strachan B, Murphy DJ. Pelvic floor morbidity at 3 years after instrumental delivery and cesarean delivery in the second stage of labor and the impact of a subsequent delivery. Am J Obstet Gynecol. 2005;192(3):789–94.

25. Murphy DJ, Liebling RE, Verity L, Swingler R, Patel R. Early maternal and neonatal morbidity associated with operative delivery in second stage of labour: a cohort study. The Lancet. 2001;358(9289):1203–7.

26. Anim-Somuah M, Smyth RM, Cyna AM, Cuthbert A. Epidural versus non-epidural or no analgesia for pain management in labour. Cochrane Db Syst Rev. 2018;2018(5):CD000331.

27. Arulkumaran S, Robson M. *Munro Kerr's Operative Obstetrics*. 13th ed. Arulkumaran S, Robson M, editors. London, UK: Elsevier; 2019. p. 320.

28. UKARCOG. ReDEFINe (Rotational DElivery at Full dIlatatioN). 2018. (RCOG National Trainees Conference). http://ukarcog.org/wp-content/uploads/2018/01/ReDEFINe-facts-and-figures-poster.pdf

29. Murphy DJ, Macleod M, Bahl R, Strachan B. A cohort study of maternal and neonatal morbidity in relation to use of sequential instruments at operative vaginal delivery. Eur J Obstet Gyn R B. 2011;156(1):41–5.

30. Tempest N, McGuinness N, Lane S, Hapangama DK. Neonatal and maternal outcomes of successful manual rotation to correct malposition of the fetal head; a retrospective and prospective observational study. PLoS one. 2017;12(5):e0176861.

31. Royal College of Obstetricians and Gynaecologists. *Consent Advice No. 11 – Operative Vaginal Birth* [Internet]. London, UK: Royal College of Obstetricians and Gynaecologists; 2010. https://www.rcog.org.uk/globalassets/documents/guidelines/ca11-15072010.pdf

32. Bellussi F, Ghi T, Youssef A et al. The use of intrapartum ultrasound to diagnose malpositions and cephalic malpresentations. Am J Obstet Gynecol. 2017;217(6):633–41.

33. Parry-Jones E. The use of Kielland's forceps. *Br J Clin Pract*. 1952;11(6):434–43.

34. Aiken AR, Aiken CE, Alberry MS, Brockelsby JC, Scott JG. Management of fetal malposition in the second stage of labor: a propensity score analysis. Am J Obstet Gynecol [Internet]. 2015;212(3):355.e1-355.e7. message:%3C20151214135424.88D364B836F@nhs-pd1e-esg009.ad1.nhs.net%3E

# Chapter 7
# Caesarean Section at Full Cervical Dilatation

Patrick O'Brien and Sadia Bhatti

## Key Learning Points

- To learn about the possible maternal and fetal complications associated with a second stage caesarean section.
- Techniques to perform safer second stage caesarean section.
- Techniques to identify and manage the fetal and maternal complications.
- Preventive measures to minimise fetal and maternal complications.

## Incidence

There are currently no precise figures for the incidence of caesarean section at full dilatation, but given that there are around 200,000 caesarean births in the UK each year with around 10% at full dilatation, it potentially affects around 20,000 births per year.[1]

According to the Royal College of Obstetricians and Gynaecologists' audit figures, around 35% of caesareans for singleton pregnancies were performed because of lack of progress in labour, of which a quarter occur at full cervical dilatation. In 55% of these cases, no attempt was made to achieve an assisted vaginal birth with either forceps or ventouse. In those where instrumental delivery was attempted, the audit found a failure rate of 35% for ventouse and 2% for forceps.[2]

# Background

Loudon et al.[3] demonstrated that over the decade from 1992 to 2001 the use of forceps fell while more deliveries were performed with the aid of ventouse; however, births attempted with the assistance of ventouse were more likely to fail. There was an increase in caesarean sections at full dilatation due to both failed attempts at instrumental birth and an increased reluctance to attempt instrumentation. Whether this is directly due to trainees' reduced working hours and therefore clinical training and experience, or whether it is simply the continuation of a trend towards a lower threshold for caesarean section, is impossible to decipher. As long ago as 2009, the Postgraduate Medical Education and Training Board (PMETB) trainees' survey[4] reported that 8.8% of trainees said that, if faced with a woman at full dilatation with a fetal malposition and station below the ischial spines, they would deliver by caesarean section, without an attempt at instrumental delivery. This survey showed that an increasing number of women were being taken to theatre at full dilatation, and that in itself may have influenced the mode of delivery by lowering the threshold for caesarean section.

# Factors Which May Predispose to caesarean Section at Full Dilatation

## Cephalopelvic Disproportion

Obstructed labour, the direct clinical consequence of cephalopelvic disproportion (CPD), is responsible for 8% of maternal deaths worldwide, according to the 2005 World Health Report of the World Health Organization.[5] The report estimates that, in the year 2000, obstructed labour complicated 4.6% of live births (a total of six million births), resulting in 42,000 maternal deaths, most in sub-Saharan Africa.

CPD occurs in a pregnancy where there is a mismatch in size between the fetal head and the maternal pelvis, resulting in 'failure of the fetus to pass safely through the birth canal for mechanical reasons'. This may be caused by the fetal head outgrowing the capacity of the maternal birth canal, or by presentation in a position or attitude that will not allow descent through the pelvis. Untreated, the consequence is obstructed labour, which can endanger the lives of both mother and fetus.

Maternal factors that predispose to CPD include contracted pelvis, pelvic exostoses and spondylolisthesis. Predisposing fetal factors include hydrocephalus, large infant, brow presentation, face presentation (mento-posterior), occipito-posterior position and deflexed head.

## Fetal Compromise

In a retrospective study of the efficacy of electronic fetal monitoring combined with fetal blood gas analysis during labour in identifying fetal compromise,[5] assisted delivery for 'fetal distress' was performed in 9% of 2,659 births. All had continuous fetal heart rate monitoring and 22% had a fetal scalp blood analysis. Assisted delivery had been performed in 53% of the infants who were acidotic at birth (umbilical artery pH < 7.20) and in 46% of those with a low Apgar score (<7). These results show that the use of continuous fetal heart rate monitoring and fetal scalp blood sampling detects fetal compromise without resulting in a high rate of assisted delivery.[6] However, there is evidence that continuous fetal monitoring does increase likelihood of interventions, including caesarean section.

## High Maternal Body Mass Index

Women with a high body mass index (BMI) are at increased risk of emergency caesarean section.[8] A meta-analysis of 33 cohort studies showed that, compared to women with a normal BMI, the OR for caesarean section (either elective or emergency) among women defined as overweight and obese was 1.46 (95% CI 1.34–1.60) and 2.05 (95% CI 1.86– 2.27), respectively.[7,8]

## Early Labour Immobilisation/Epidural

It has been postulated that epidural anaesthesia may increase the risk of emergency caesarean section, particularly caesarean section at full dilatation because of impaired ability to push in the second stage. However, a Cochrane Systematic Review of 21 RCTs (n = 6,664 women) compared epidural (all forms) versus non-epidural or no analgesia. The second stage of labour was significantly longer for women with epidural analgesia (10 trials) and the incidence of instrumental birth was higher for this group compared with women with non-epidural analgesia or no analgesia. Epidural analgesia was also associated with an increased incidence of oxytocin augmentation, maternal hypotension, maternal fever over 38°C and urinary retention. However, there was no significant difference in the caesarean section rate between the epidural and non-epidural groups.[9]

# Preparation

## Appropriate Place

An operating theatre with good lighting is a basic prerequisite. Ensure good aseptic technique (because of the increased risk of infection associated with caesarean section at full dilation) and adequate (preferably experienced) assistance and scrub staff. The most senior obstetrician available should be present in case of difficult delivery or repair. An experienced midwife or doctor should be in theatre in case vaginal disimpaction of the fetal head is required.

## Analgesia

Prior to the procedure, discuss with the anaesthetist the likelihood of difficult delivery. The anaesthetist should be prepared to administer drugs that induce uterine relaxation or to adjust the height or inclination of the operating table, if required. Request in advance that, as well as the oxytocin bolus, an oxytocin infusion should be commenced as soon as the baby is delivered (or carbetocin may be used as an alternative to an oxytocin bolus and infusion).

## Consent and WHO Checklist

As well as the usual risks of infection, haemorrhage, thrombosis and bladder damage, the consent form should document the increased risk of blood transfusion associated with full dilatation caesarean section. During the WHO checklist procedure, make the theatre staff aware that this is a full dilatation caesarean section and of the grade of urgency. Give clear advice about the possible complications, including potentially difficult delivery and haemorrhage.

## Examination in the Theatre

In women in whom the full dilatation caesarean section is not preceded by a failed instrumental delivery, abdominal and vaginal examination is mandatory before proceeding to caesarean section as the findings can change quickly in the second stage of labour. This does not cause any significant delay; it can be performed at the time of insertion of the urinary catheter.

## Vaginal Disinfection

A Cochrane Review in 2018 showed that vaginal disinfection with povidone-iodine or chlorhexidine immediately prior to caesarean section probably reduces the risk of post-operative endometritis, and the benefit is greatest in those already in labour or with ruptured membranes.[10]

## Disimpaction

Before making the skin incision, ensure that an experienced member of staff (midwife or doctor) is allocated to flex and push the head up vaginally, if required. Advise them to use their whole hand, and not just a few fingers, in order to distribute the force more evenly and minimise the risk of trauma to the fetal skull. They should be instructed to flex and then disimpact the fetal head. Check that this person is ready and explain to the theatre runners that they may need to help this person access the vagina (by lifting the sterile drapes and flexing the woman's legs). A fetal pillow may be used if part of a continuous audit or research study, in line with NICE guidance.[11,12]

## Neonatologist

Ensure that the neonatologist is aware of the type of caesarean section. (S)he should be present in theatre for the delivery as in second stage caesarean there is often an element of fetal compromise and always the possibility of a difficult delivery.

## Prophylactic Antibiotics

Prophylactic intravenous antibiotics should be given for all caesarean sections, elective and emergency, in line with NICE guidance.[9] As the risk of infection is increased in second stage compared with first stage or elective caesarean sections, this is of utmost importance. The antibiotics should be given before the skin incision as this reduces the risk of infection by 48% compared to when the antibiotics are given after clamping of the umbilical cord.[13]

**Lower the height of the operating table or use a step (see below).**

# Surgical Technique

## Uterine Incision

- **The Pfannenstiel incision:** this was introduced in 1900 and is widely used for caesarean section. It has excellent cosmetic results, a low incidence of wound breakdown and allows for early ambulation. The initial incision is made cleanly through the skin, just within the pubic hairline and slightly convex towards the pubis. The fat is incised down to the rectus sheath and the aponeurosis of the external oblique muscle. Short incisions are made on the rectus sheath on either side of the midline and then extended for the full length using scissors. The upper and lower edges of the incision are then grasped in turn, and the underlying muscle is separated from the rectus sheath by both blunt and sharp dissection. Caution must be taken to avoid injury to the ilioinguinal and iliohypogastric nerves when extending into the external and internal oblique muscles.

- **The Joel Cohen incision**: this is a straight transverse incision, positioned slightly higher than the Pfannenstiel. The subcutaneous tissue is not sharply divided. The anterior rectus sheath is incised in the midline for 3 cm and extended laterally digitally, but the muscles are not separated from the sheath. The peritoneum is bluntly opened in a transverse direction.

The Pfannenstiel and Joel Cohen techniques have been compared.[14] Less fever, pain, blood loss, analgesic requirements and post-operative morbidity, as well as shorter operating time, were demonstrated in the Joel Cohen incision group.

## Bladder Reflection

As there is an increased risk of extension of the uterine incision during delivery at a full dilation caesarean section, the bladder should be reflected well down, both centrally and laterally (most extensions are at the lateral angles of the incision).

## Identification of Lower Uterine Segment

Care must be taken to identify correctly the true level of the lower uterine segment. Use the utero-vesical reflection of the visceral peritoneum as a landmark, as the bladder may be higher than expected when the cervix is fully dilated.

## Opening the Uterine Cavity

After reflecting the bladder well down, make a careful uterine incision. Make this incision a little higher than usual (but still in the lower segment) to ensure that you are clear of the fully dilated cervix and vagina. The lower segment is likely to be thin, so incise carefully so as not to cut the baby. Having made a superficial incision, attempt to enter the uterus using a finger rather than the knife. Keep the initial incision small; there may be some benefit in making it U-shaped. If the lower segment is very thin, consider extending the initial incision laterally with a pair of scissors in a U–shape (Figure 7.1). This creates an adequate opening for delivery while reducing the chances of an uncontrolled tear caused by stretching the opening manually. It also helps to direct the incision (and any tear) away from the uterine arteries which ascend the lateral aspect of the uterus.

As you open the uterus be aware that, as the fetal head is low in the pelvis, the fetal arm may present at the uterine incision. So, as you open the uterus, be prepared to prevent the arm from delivering first. If the arm does deliver, it will make delivery of the rest of the baby very difficult. In this situation, the arm should be replaced into the uterus (and held there) before attempting to deliver the head.

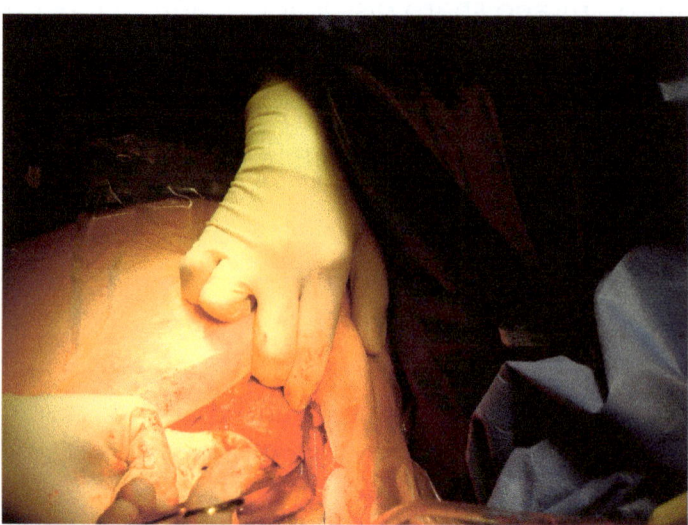

**Figure 7.1** Extending the uterine incision.

If not extending the uterine incision with the scissors, the index fingers of each hand are used to do so, extending the incision laterally and upwards along the path of least resistance so that the presenting part can be delivered. When there is difficulty in delivering the presenting part, an extension of the transverse incision in the shape of a 'J' is better than an inverted 'T' as it will heal better and is therefore considered stronger.

## Previous Abdominal Surgery

In women who have had previous abdominal surgery, anticipate that entry and bladder reflection may be more difficult, and ensure that senior help is available. When the bladder is adherent, take time (assuming there is no urgency to deliver the baby) to ensure adequate bladder dissection and reflection. If the bladder is not adequately reflected before delivery, and there is a significant extension of the uterine incision during delivery, it can present major difficulty. First, the adherent bladder may tear with the uterus. Second, even if the bladder is not damaged, it may be necessary to dissect it free of the torn lower segment in order to gain access to the uterine tear. This dissection will be far more difficult than it would have been prior to making the uterine incision (and the woman will now be bleeding so there will be more urgency).

## Delivery of Fetal Head

Follow these steps:

1. Introduce a hand below the baby's head.
2. Flex the baby's head. If the position is occipito-anterior (OA), this is usually easy. If the position is occipito-posterior (OP), a common cause of obstructed labour, this may be more difficult. Make sure that you introduce your hand

around the baby's head until you can feel the occiput; only then should you try to flex it.

3. Disimpact the head (see below).

4. Deliver the head through the uterine incision.

<u>Do not</u> skip any of these four steps; it will make delivery more difficult and extension of the uterine incision more likely. For example, if you try to disimpact an OP head before flexing it, it may result in further deflexion but no disimpaction. If you try to deliver the baby's head before disimpacting, it will lead to extension of the uterine incision.

## Lower the Height of the Operating Table

Or consider using a step, depending on individual height. The aim is to have the table low enough that you can keep your arm straight during delivery of the head. If the head is very impacted, this makes manipulation and disimpaction easier.

## Disimpacting the Fetal Head

Your hand should be below the head at the occiput. Attempt to disimpact only after you have successfully flexed the head, particularly when it is in an OP position. Apply traction in the maternal long axis, that is, towards the mother's head. Do not attempt to deliver the baby's head at this stage. A 'suction' sound is often heard as the pressure seal is broken (Figure 7.2).

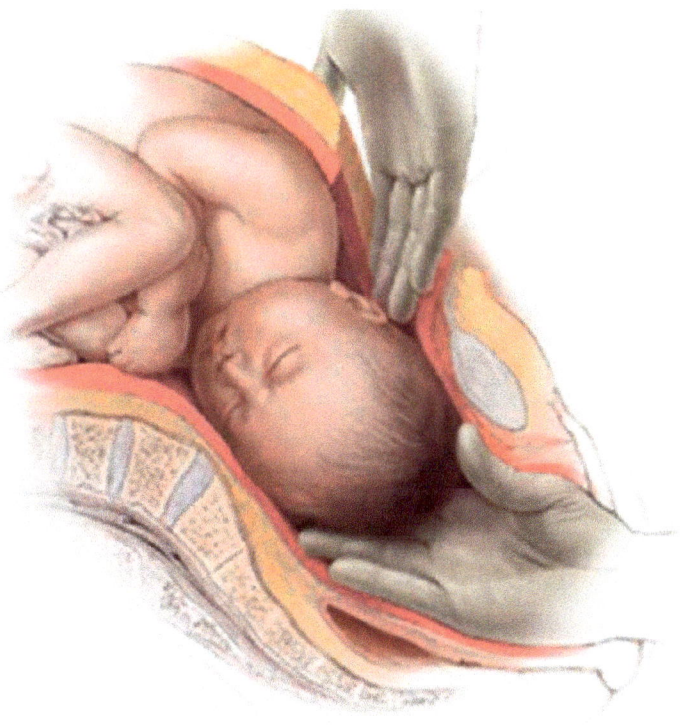

**Figure 7.2** Disimpacting the fetal head.

### Measures to be Taken if There is Difficulty Disimpacting the Fetal Head

At this stage, if the surgeon has difficulty disimpacting the baby's head from above (and if a fetal pillow has not already been used) the assistant (who should be standing by) can be asked to push up the baby's head vaginally. This should be done by flexing the fetal head and then disimpacting it into the pelvis. Pressure should be spread over as many fingers as possible, in order to minimise the risk of trauma to the fetal skull. Ideally, this person should introduce her or his whole hand into the vagina. In addition, if necessary, the scrubbed assistant can help by applying pressure on the fetal shoulders (again pushing towards the mother's head) which are often at the level of the uterine incision in this situation.

A uterine relaxant can be administered by the anaesthetist. One option is sublingual glyceryl trinitrite (GTN, two sprays). GTN sprays can be repeated at five-minute intervals and take one to two minutes to work. GTN is contra-indicated in hypovolaemia, raised intracranial pressure and nitrate sensitivity.

Tilting the operating table head down may aid disimpaction (although may be uncomfortable for a woman who is awake, so is not usually done unless other measures have failed).

### Reverse Breech Delivery

Delivering the fetus as a breech is an alternative when disimpacting the head proves impossible (Figure 7.3). Schwake et al.[15] showed that this technique is feasible and carries a low risk of maternal and neonatal morbidity. Previous studies examining the reverse breech manoeuvre during second stage

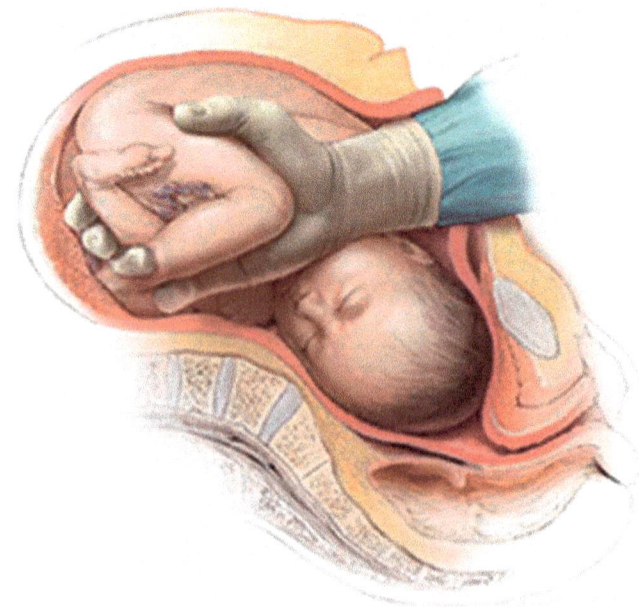

**Figure 7.3** If disimpacting the head proves impossible, the alternative way is to grasp a leg and deliver the fetus as breech.

caesarean section have found this method preferable to the abdomino-vaginal approach – the push method.[16,17] Inadvertent extension of the uterine incision and maternal postpartum complications were more prevalent in the push method than the reverse breech approach.

# Maternal Complications

## Extension of the Uterine Incision

Extension of the uterine incision most commonly occurs from one or both angles. In this situation, exteriorising the uterus is very helpful. It allows better visualisation of the angles and any tears, and it makes access for the repair much easier. By placing the uterine arteries under tension, it also reduces the amount of bleeding. Always advise the anaesthetist in advance when you need to exteriorise the uterus, as it may make the woman uncomfortable and may cause some vagal stimulation, leading to the woman feeling faint or nauseous.

- A second assistant is valuable to help provide better exposure when there are suspected extensions
- If required, call for help of adequate seniority early
- Identify the apex at each end of the uterine incision
- Ensure that the bladder is reflected well down, that is, clear of the uterine incision and any tears
- Identify the ureters, particularly when the tear extends infero-laterally (which is common).

If there is significant bleeding and difficult access, it is preferable to begin the repair with a blunt Vicryl no.1 suture, as it reduces the chances of a needle-stick injury to the surgeon or (more commonly) to the assistant. However, when the tissues are very friable, a sharp needle may be more appropriate for precise placement of sutures.

Occasionally, when the apex of a tear descending deep into the pelvis cannot be reached, the first suture should be placed safely as low as possible in the tear, leaving the tied end of the suture long. Once tied, the two ends of the suture can then be used to pull upwards on the tear; then another suture can be placed lower down. In this way, the suture can be advanced stepwise until the apex of the tear is reached.

### Extension into the Broad Ligament

This possibility should always be borne in mind and checked for. The accumulation of blood may not initially be obvious. If on palpation there is suspicion of a broad ligament haematoma, the broad ligament should be opened. Pressure and Vicryl 0 or 2/0 can be used to achieve haemostasis.

## Cervical or High Vaginal Lacerations

An extension of the uterine incision may be directed downwards and involve the cervix (which is fully dilated so often close to the uterine incision) and even vagina (which at full dilatation is continuous with the lower segment). In this situation, it sometimes proves impossible to achieve complete repair from above (abdominally). In this case, the woman may need a combined abdominal and vaginal repair in the lithotomy position with two experienced operators, one at the abdominal incision and the other operating vaginally. There is a significant risk of ureteric (or even urethral) involvement; if this occurs, the urology team should be involved.

## Damage to Bladder or Ureter

This is more likely in situations of downward extension of a uterine tear, either laterally or anteriorly. Accidental involvement of a ureter in a suture is more likely when the anatomy is distorted by the tear, particularly when there is poor visualisation of the operative field due to bleeding or because it is deep in the pelvis. Exteriorisation of the uterus will help to avoid such trauma. Careful identification of the ureters and bladder is essential, and there should always be a high index of suspicion in such situations. If any damage to the bladder or ureters is detected (or suspected), a urology opinion should be sought. Methylene blue dye is injected into the bladder via the urinary catheter to identify any leak. This dye should be available in all obstetric theatres.

## Post-Partum Haemorrhage and Blood Transfusion

These are more common because of an increased likelihood of uterine atony and trauma.[18]

## Further Surgery

bladder repair, hysterectomy internal iliac artery ligation, or repair of genital tract tears and extensions are more common.[18]

## Sepsis

Sepsis is more common following emergency than elective caesarean section, particularly following caesarean at full dilatation.[18] Vaginal disinfection with povidone-iodine or chlorhexidine before commencing the operation, and IV prophylactic antibiotics, which should be given prior to the uterine incision, reduce this risk.[10,13]

## Addmission to Intensive Care Unit (ICU)

Admission to ICU is more common because of the complications mentioned above, in particular haemorrhage and sepsis.[18]

# Fetal Complications

## Skull Fracture Due to Impacted Head

Skull fracture may occasionally occur during difficult disimpaction of the fetal head during a second stage, or late first stage, caesarean section. Increasingly, women who fail to deliver vaginally are undergoing caesarean section in the late first and second stage of labour, when difficulty in delivering the impacted fetal head is most commonly reported. Fetal trauma following impacted head at caesarean section is an increasing cause of litigation in the UK and elsewhere.

The average maternal BMI is also increasing. Pregnant women with a high BMI are more likely to undergo induction or augmentation of labour, and have an increased risk of caesarean section in the late first and second stage of labour, which increases the risk of intrapartum complications associated with impaction of the fetal head.[7]

## Limb Fractures

Limb fracture is uncommon during delivery of a term baby but more likely in a difficult preterm delivery. Studies have shown that there is no increase in the incidence of fractures in reverse breech deliveries during caesarean section.[16,17]

## Advanced Resuscitation

Studies have demonstrated that compared with caesarean delivery at less than full cervical dilatation, women undergoing caesarean at full dilatation were 1.5 times more likely to deliver an infant with perinatal asphyxia and requiring advanced resuscitation. However, no differences were seen in the rates of neonatal trauma, low 5-minute Apgar score or neonatal sepsis.[19]

# Prevention of Complications of Second Stage caesarean Section

## Training

### Desperate Debra® (Simulated Training)

The Desperate Debra® (Figure 7.4) simulates the abdomen, uterus and fetus of a birthing mother, and has a mechanism to replicate an impacted fetal head.

Education and training towards gaining the following skills are possible:

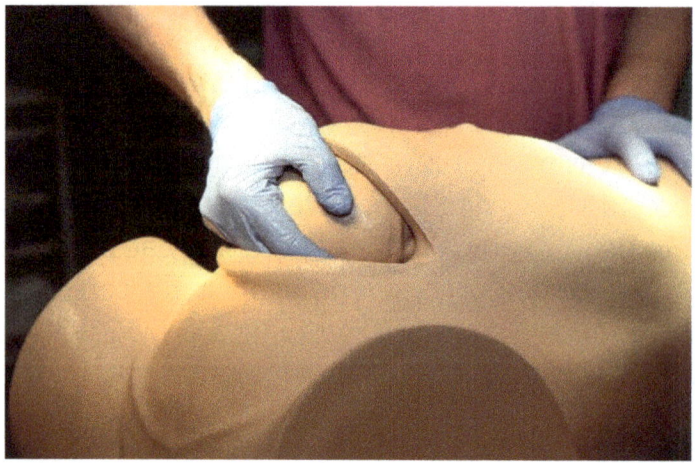

**Figure 7.4** The Desperate Debra® model allows the simulation of disimpacting and delivering the fetal head. Photo courtesy: Adam Rouilly.

- Successful delivery of an impacted fetal head at caesarean section (with adjustable degrees of difficulty)
- Vaginal examination in advanced labour
- Identification of fetal head position and variable degrees of flexion and asynclitism – the model has palpable fontanelles and sutures

### Interactive Courses

### Labour Ward Supervision and Early Senior Involvement

Labour ward supervision to improve rotational instrumental delivery skills and experience will help to reduce the incidence of full dilatation caesarean section.[21]

# Debriefing

Good communication with the woman and her birth partner throughout the delivery is essential. When the obstetrician is preoccupied with a difficult delivery, the supporting midwife or anaesthetist should take on this role. After the delivery, preferably the same day or the following day at the latest, it is the duty of the most senior obstetrician involved to debrief the couple about the events around delivery. Second stage caesarean sections can be associated with a series of events occurring in rapid succession and the parents can be left confused about exactly what happened and why. It is important that the clinicians involved take the time to explain the events clearly to the parents so that they fully understand what happened and the reasons for any difficulties. The possibility of vaginal birth (or not) for future births should also be discussed at this stage.

# Documentation

It is the responsibility of the operating surgeons and anaesthetists to ensure that all relevant documentation is completed. This will include the operating notes and perhaps an adverse incident reporting form, and any relevant proformas in use in that unit (e.g. for postpartum haemorrhage). Ensure that correct timings of events are recorded; it is valuable to designate a scribe whose role is to document events and timings in real time during the procedure. Where indicated, illustrative diagrams of any extensive tears and repairs should be considered, as these may be helpful in the management of future pregnancies. Always document the position of the baby's head when the uterus was opened; this may be very valuable information when deciding whether aiming for a vaginal birth (VBAC) in the next pregnancy is feasible.

| Points to remember | | |
|---|---|---|
| Pre-operative | Be prepared<br>Lower the table<br>Disinfect the vagina | Get appropriate help<br>Consider use of fetal pillow<br>Allocate someone to be ready to push up on the fetal head vaginally |
| Intra-operative | Stay calm<br><br>Communicate with your anaesthetist<br>Reflect bladder well down before uterine incision<br>Consider extending uterine incision with scissors<br><br>Always flex the head well before attempting to disimpact<br><br>Exteriorise the uterus if there is a significant tear or heavy bleeding | Don't fight the uterine cavity<br>Compression pressure on bleeders not the suction<br>Uterine incision a little higher than usual<br><br>Watch for, and prevent, delivery of a presenting arm when opening the uterus<br>Always disimpact the head completely from the pelvis before attempting to deliver the head<br>Get urological support if there is suspicion of damage to the urinary tract |

(cont.)

| Points to remember | | |
| --- | --- | --- |
| Post-operative | Be prepared for postpartum haemorrhage<br>Sepsis<br>Check for perineal trauma, if appropriate, e.g. failed instrumental delivery | Antibiotics as required<br>Debrief the parents<br>Documentation |

# References

1.  Office for National Statistics. UK statistics for caesarean sections, Births in England and Wales 2009. www.statistics.gov.uk/statbase; ISD Scotland www.isdscot.org

2.  Thomas J, Paranjothy S. Royal College of Obstetricians and Gynaecologists Clinical Effectiveness Support Unit. *The National Sentinel caesarean Section Audit Report*. London: RCOG Press, 2001.

3.  Loudon JA, Groom KM, Hinkson L, Harrington D, Paterson-Brown S. Changing trends in operative delivery performed at full dilatation over a 10-year period. J Obstet Gynaecol. 2010 ;30(4):370–5. doi: 10.3109/01443611003628411. PMID: 20455720.

4.  Postgraduate Medical Education Training Board. 2008–2009 Trainees Survey. www.gmc-uk.org/ National_Training_Surveys_2008_09_20090929.pdf_30512348.pdf

5.  World Health Organization. Make every mother and child count. The World Health Report 2005. whqlibdoc.who.int/whr/2005/9241562900

6.  Van Den Berg P, Schmidt S, Gesche J, Saling E. Fetal distress and the condition of the newborn using cardiotocography and fetal blood analysis during labour. BJOG 1987; 94: 72–5. https:// doi.org/10.1111/j.1471-0528.1987.tb02256.x

7.  Zhang J, Bricker L, Wray S, Quenby S. Poor uterine contractility in obese women. BJOG 2007;114:343–8.

8.  Denison FC, Aedla NR, Keag O et al., on behalf of the Royal College of Obstetricians and Gynaecologists. Care of Women with Obesity in Pregnancy. Green-top Guideline No. 72. *BJOG* 2018. www.rcog.org.uk/files/rcogcorp/CMACERCOGJointGuideline

9.  National Institute for Health and Care Excellence. Intrapartum Care (NG235). London: NICE; 2023. nice.org.uk/nicemedia/live/11837/36275/36275

10. Haas DM, Morgan S, Contreras K et al. Vaginal preparation with antiseptic solution before cesarean section for preventing postoperative infections. *Cochrane Database Syst Rev* 2018;**30**: CD007892.doi:10.1002/14651858.CD007892.pub6

11. Seal SL, Dey A, Barman SC et al. Randomized controlled trial of elevation of the fetal head with a fetal pillow during cesarean delivery at full cervical dilatation. Int J Gynaecol Obstet. 2016;133:178–82. doi: 10.1016/j.ijgo.2015.09.019. Epub 2016 Jan 15. PMID: 26868074.

12. Di Girolamo R, Galliani C, Buca D, Liberati M, D'Antonio F. Outcomes of second stage cesarean section following the use of a fetal head elevation device: a systematic review and meta-analysis. Eur J Obstet Gynecol Reprod Biol. 2021. doi: https://doi.org/10.1016/j.ejogrb.2021.04.043

13. Kittur, ND, McMullen, KM, Russo, AJ et al. Long-term effect of infection prevention practices and case mix on cesarean surgical site infections. Obstet Gynecol : 2012;120:246–51.

14. Karanth KL, Sathish N. Review of advantages of Joel-Cohen surgical abdominal incision in caesarean section: a basic science perspective. Med J Malaysia. 2010;65:204–208.

15. Schwake D Petchenkin L, Younis JS. Reverse breech extraction in cases of second stage caesarean section. J Obstet Gynaecol 2012;32:548–51.

16. Fasubaa OB, Ezechi OC, Orji EO et al. Delivery of the impacted head of the fetus at caesarean section after prolonged obstructed labour: a randomized comparative study of two methods. J Obstet Gynaecol 2002;22:375–8.

17. Chopra S, Bagga R, Keepanasseril A et al. Disengagement of the deeply engaged fetal head during cesarean section in advanced labor: conventional method versus reverse breech extraction. Acta Obstet Gynecol Scan 2009;88:1163–6.

18. McKelvey A, Ashe R, McKenna D, Roberts R. caesarean section in the second stage of labour: a retrospective review of obstetric setting and morbidity. J Obstet Gynaecol. 2010 ;30(3):264–7. doi:10.3109/01443610903572109.PMID:20373928.

19. Allen VM, O' Connell CM, Baskett TF. Maternal and perinatal morbidity of caesarean delivery at full cervical dilatation compared with caesarean delivery in the first stage of labour. Br J Obstet Gynaecol 2005;112:986–90.

20. Desperate Debra® – Impacted Fetal Head Simulator. www.adam-rouilly.co.uk/productdetails

21. Spencer C, Murphy D, Bewley S. caesarean section in the second stage of labour. BMJ 2006; 333:613–4.

# Chapter 8

# Medico-Legal Aspects of Assisted Vaginal Birth (AVB)

Milena Petrovic, Dimitrios Siassakos and Derek Tuffnell

## Key Learning Points

■ To identify the areas for potential litigation related to AVB to inform training.

■ To define effective strategies to minimise risks related to AVB for both mother and baby and improve overall quality of care.

## Introduction

Maternity claims represent the highest value and second highest number of clinical negligence claims reported to NHS Resolution. The three most frequent categories of claim were those relating to **management of labour** (14.05%), **caesarean section** (13.24%) and **cerebral palsy** (10.65%). Two of these categories, namely cerebral palsy and management of labour, along with CTG interpretation, were also the most expensive and together accounted for approximately 70% of the total figure of £3.1 billion, paid out on or expected to be paid, for all maternity claims.[1]

Review of the claims on the NHS Resolution database with an incident date between 1 April 2000 and 31 March 2010 identified 160 claims involving **assisted vaginal delivery**: 88 of these relate to forceps deliveries; 42 to Ventouse deliveries; and in 30 claims the instrument was not stated. The estimated total value of the claims was £94 million.[1]

# Assisted Vaginal Birth: Potential Areas of Litigation

AVB is an alternative for women to achieve vaginal delivery when spontaneous delivery is not imminent or needs to be expedited. Although considered safe, when serious adverse events occur, such as traumatic birth injury, shoulder dystocia, cerebral palsy and perinatal death, there are medico-legal implications.[2]

## Areas of Litigation in Assisted Vaginal Birth

### Insufficient information provided

■ Insufficient information about management options, procedure explanation and time for decision and/or discussion prior to obtaining the consent

■ Minimal, unclear or no communication with the patient and birth partner (before, throughout and after the procedure).

### Delay in deciding to intervene or delay in achieving birth

### Criteria for safe assisted vaginal birth are not met or judged incorrectly

■ Inappropriate choice of location for safe assisted vaginal birth

■ Inappropriate choice of instrument

■ Inappropriate application and use of instrument

■ Failure to anticipate possible complications and timely request for help

■ Failure to timely recognise that the procedure needs to be abandoned.

### The consequences of these deficiencies are either adverse maternal or fetal outcome:

■ Fetal hypoxia/fetal trauma

■ Maternal trauma (mostly perineal)/haemorrhage/psychological.

The 'enemy' of litigation is patient-centred yet evidence-based practice, good communication and appropriate documentation. 'You do not get sued for what you have done but for what you have written' is not correct. On some occasions courts might accept the evidence from women and their families over what is documented in the medical notes but, with continuity of care and candour, complications may never end up as a complaint or in court.

# Preventing Adverse Outcomes and Litigation

## Reasonable Antenatal Information

The NHS Litigation Authority's 'Ten Years of Maternity Claims' report has shown that the majority of claims were with patients who were not identified as high risk.[1] Hence, the importance of accurate and timely information about what to expect during labour and giving birth, even when the pregnancy is not classified as high risk, is a step forward in minimising risks of complications and medico-legal implications.

Information about AVB should ideally be included in antenatal classes and supported with high-quality information leaflets (e.g. RCOG Assisted Vaginal Birth, Patient Information, April 2020), as discussions during the labour often may be time-limited and constrained by pain and stress.

For the practising obstetrician, it means that any opportunity to discuss AVB should be used wisely. It is particularly important to discuss and dispel myths, and fears based on the experiences of others. In the experience of the authors, most of the cases where women decline choices medically indicated and preferred (for example, refusing forceps at full dilatation with the vertex below the spines) are the result of a lack of information and/or misinformation. The misunderstandings are usually, if not always, resolved with appropriate information discussed with a suitably experienced accoucheur – in the instance above, by explaining that caesarean section at full dilatation has higher risks for both mother and fetus, but becomes the only option if a trial of AVB fails first. Such fears rarely emerge out of the blue in labour and can be elicited and addressed well in advance if only women are given the chance to express their concerns and ask questions at every opportunity.

However, claims often arise because it is indicated there was a failure to explain the AVB procedure and offer the option of caesarean section, when the decision to deliver is made. This is challenging in emergency situations; however it is important that the consent form includes details and the risks of all the procedures, not just caesarean section risks with the risks of severe perineal and fetal trauma not mentioned – as is often seen on written consent forms for 'trial' of assisted birth.

## Reduce Need for AVB

There are numerous evidence-based recommendations[3,4] to increase the chance of spontaneous vaginal birth, including:

■ **Continuous support during labour**

Continuous support for women during childbirth has been shown to increase the likelihood of spontaneous vaginal birth (26 trials; $n$ = 15,858; risk ratio [RR] 1.08, 95% CI 1.04–1.12) and reduce the likelihood of assisted vaginal birth (RR 0.90, 95% CI 0.85–0.96), particularly when the carer is not a member of staff.[3]

■ **Position during the first stage of labour**

It is important to promote and support mobility. Squatting increases the transverse diameters of the mid-pelvis and the antero-posterior diameters of the lower pelvis, promoting the cardinal movements of labour.[5]

■ **Position during first stage of labour**

☐ lying down lateral positions rather than upright positions, for women using epidural

☐ upright or lateral, for women not using epidural

The use of any upright or lateral position in the second stage of labour, compared with supine or lithotomy positions, is associated with a reduction in assisted births in women not using epidural analgesia (21 trials; $n$ = 6,481; RR 0.75, 95% CI 0.66 to –0.86).[3]

■ **Delayed pushing for one to two hours in nulliparous women with epidural analgesia**

A meta-analysis demonstrated that nulliparous women with epidurals are likely to have fewer rotational or mid-pelvic operative interventions when pushing is delayed for one to two hours or until they have a strong urge to push (RR 0.59, 95% CI 0.36–0.98), although a more recent meta-analysis concluded that when the analysis is restricted to high-quality studies, the effect was smaller and did not reach statistical significance.[3]

■ **Ensure the bladder is empty** before commencing active pushing

■ **Encouragement[4] – 'coaching'**, by an experienced accoucheur, if pushing is ineffective or if requested by the woman

■ **Use of oxytocin for nulliparous women[4]** if contractions are inadequate at the onset of second stage

## Informed Consent

### Shared decision-making and consent are fundamental to good medical practice.[6]

The consent process should always have been an informed and meaningful dialogue rather than a one-sided decision. The implication of the 2015 *Montgomery* ruling has been to detail the legal expectation as to the nature of the way in which information is shared. There is a clearer requirement to ensure women are aware of the options in terms of management and the risks and benefits of each approach. The determination as to which risks should be explained are those which the woman would consider material.

In practice, this means that every healthcare professional must:[7]

■ Clearly outline the recommended management strategies and procedures to their patient, including the risks, benefits and implications of potential treatment options in a timely manner – this may include antenatal counselling about labour and delivery issues

■ Discuss any alternative treatments

■ Discuss the consequences of not performing any treatment or intervention; ideally this should be discussed with more than one accoucheurs if time permits

■ Ensure patients have access to high-quality information to aid their decision-making

■ Give patients adequate time to reflect before making a decision

■ Check patients have fully understood their options and the implications, acknowledging the challenges of labour (e.g. pain, emergencies)

■ Document the above process in the patient's record

Ideally, written consent should always be obtained. More importantly, the risks and benefits material to each patient, by nature of their high risk or high concern for the patient and her family, should be discussed and should be documented. This is clearly much more challenging in an emergency situation. However, for procedures in the birth room and in the emergency situation verbal consent witnessed by another healthcare professional is sufficient and considered to be in the best interest of the woman or baby.[8] In some instances (category 1 urgency) a signed consent form waved in front of a stressed and rapidly moved (e.g. to theatre) woman is anything but informed consent, and a few sentences by a calm experienced caregiver are more appropriate.

Consent during the labour has to be taken with special consideration, particularly if women are in pain or under the influence of narcotic analgesics. Also, for women with limited English language skills, an approved translation service should be provided. In such instances, discussing in advance with an interpreter (for example upon admission and initial review on labour ward, in addition to antenatal discussions) any interventions and complications that may be required, including AVB and its risks and benefits, is important and recommended. Whereas discussion in advance of interventions might be perceived as a prediction that they will be needed, which might create some apprehension, it is preferable to the scenario where interventions occur without sufficiently informed consent. It is likely to be difficult to obtain appropriate informed consent later, should an emergency need arise.

**Assisted vaginal delivery consent** should include:[9]

- ■ Serious risks

  - ☐ Maternal: third- and fourth-degree tear (1–4:100 with vacuum, 8–12:100 with forceps), extensive or significant vaginal/vulval tear (1:10 with vacuum, 1:5 with forceps)

  - ☐ Fetal: subgaleal haematoma (3–6:1,000; particularly with vacuum), intracranial haemorrhage (5–15:10,000), facial nerve palsy (permanent is rare <1:1,000; associated with forceps), skull fracture (rare)

- ■ Frequent risks

  - ☐ Maternal: PPH (1–4:10), vaginal tear/abrasion (very common, >1:10), anal sphincter/voiding dysfunction. However, it is worth mentioning that these also occur with spontaneous vaginal birth

  - ☐ Fetal: temporary forceps marks on face/cup marking on the scalp (very common, >1:10, resolve spontaneously), cephalhaematoma (1–12:100, it can occur with spontaneous vaginal birth as well), facial or scalp lacerations (1:10). Neonatal jaundice/hyperbilirubinaemia (5–15:100) can also be discussed if time allows or the mother enquires

  - ☐ Both – risk of shoulder dystocia or conversion to caesarean section (CS)

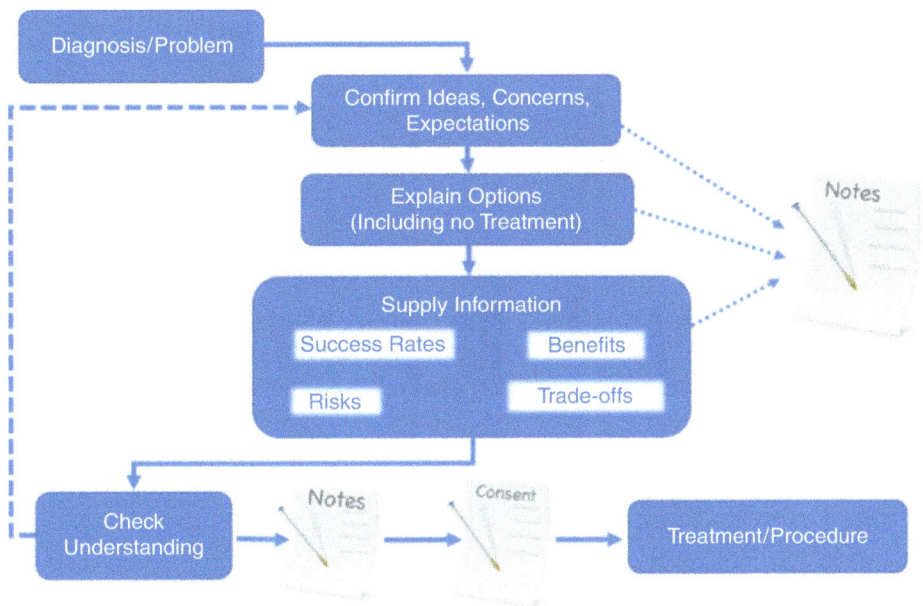

**Figure 8.1** Ideal consent process.
Adopted from RCOG Model
Consent Process.[8]

- Any extra procedure which may become necessary during the procedure
  - ☐ Manual rotation prior to vacuum/forceps assisted delivery
  - ☐ Rotation with instruments
  - ☐ Episiotomy (5–6:10 with vacuum, 9:10 with forceps delivery)
  - ☐ Manoeuvres for shoulders dystocia – important to discuss well in advance with women who have a high risk (diabetes, macrosomia)
  - ☐ Repair of perineal tear
  - ☐ Blood transfusion
  - ☐ caesarean section

The RCOG guidance on **Assisted Vaginal Delivery Consent** includes appropriate lay terminology for describing the risks above.

Whereas some complications are well described and are not always preventable, severe and multiple injuries can be criticised particularly if associated with other indicators of excessive force – for example concurrent permanent facial palsy, debilitating eye injury, and descriptions of using the knee on the bed for counter-traction.

It is important to note that not every single risk, including those not mentioned above, can be discussed in detail on every single occasion. As a minimum, the risks discussed should include those that are material because of their high risk (for example shoulder dystocia in a woman with diabetes), or their high 'value' to the individual parent (because of concern, experience, interest, etc.)

Risk is based on clinical knowledge and individual circumstances, and relative value must be elicited through open and honest discussion.

## Safest Mode of Delivery

Decision on mode of delivery in an emergency situation requires situation awareness, timely anticipation of possible, especially serious, complications, and respect of the woman's wishes and values. Common dilemmas include:

- Abnormal CTG spectrum
- AVB versus CS
- Subsequent instrument use versus CS

### Abnormal CTG

The decision-delivery interval should be appropriate to the CTG.

An abnormal CTG is an indication for rapid delivery, which might be necessary within 30 minutes, or in some instances much faster, for example if there is a prolonged deceleration/bradycardia.

Birth in the room should usually be achievable in about 15 minutes from the decision but appropriate care needs to be taken. If transfer to theatre is required for an AVB, it should be classified in urgency terms in the same way as an emergency caesarean section and birth is expected to be achieved within 30 minutes or less. With bradycardia, a decision and transfer to theatre should be completed within 9 minutes, with birth as soon after as is safe for maternal well-being.

During a trial in theatre, anaesthesia should be sufficient for immediate conversion to caesarean section. If AVB fails in theatre, the birth should be achieved as soon as possible. The aim is for 'measured haste'. If AVB has precipitated a bradycardia then birth should be achieved in less than 10 minutes from the onset of the bradycardia.

No specific CTG abnormality is an absolute indication for preferring CS over AVB and vice versa. In the hands of an experienced accoucheur, a skilful rotational ventouse procedure or Kielland's forceps birth might be both faster and safer than a caesarean. At the same time, persisting with a clearly failed attempt at AVB long after the onset of a prolonged deceleration/bradycardia increases the risk of poor neonatal outcome; and further pulls with an unsuccessful instrument may worsen the maternal condition and fetal scalp oedema and impaction.

## Assisted Vaginal Birth versus caesarean Section

The risks of caesarean section in the second stage are well-documented – a caesarean birth in the second stage of labour is associated with a significantly increased risk of major obstetric haemorrhage, prolonged hospital stay and admission of the baby to the neonatal unit compared with completed assisted vaginal birth.[10]

## Subsequent Instrument Use versus caesarean Section

The use of sequential instruments is associated with an increased risk of serious neonatal morbidity and maternal anal sphincter injury. Careful balance is required between the risks of a full dilatation caesarean section following failed vacuum extraction with the risks of forceps delivery following failed vacuum extraction. It would not be appropriate to apply forceps for a 'failed' ventouse if there has been little or no descent. Whereas the risks of a caesarean section at full dilatation are substantial, they would be compounded if a clearly failed attempt at AVB is protracted beyond three pulls, unless delivery is imminent: head at the perineum – outlet.[3]

## Ensure Assisted Vaginal Birth Is Indicated

Indications for AVB are described in detail in Chapter 2.

There is no absolute indication for AVB and case-specific clinical judgement is necessary at all times. The threshold to intervene may be lower where additional maternal/fetal risk factors coexist.

Similarly, many contra-indications are relative (e.g. suspected fetal bleeding disorders, predisposition to fetal fracture, maternal blood-borne viral infections), and the risks have to be balanced with the risks of the alternatives. There may be considerable risks if the fetal head has to be delivered abdominally from deep in the pelvis (+2 and below).

Forceps extraction is contra-indicated before full dilatation of the cervix.

The vacuum extractor is contra-indicated with a face presentation and for <32 weeks' gestation.

## Safest Place for Assisted Vaginal Birth or When to Do a Trial?

Non-rotational low and outlet AVB has a high likelihood of success and hence the majority can safely be performed in a birth room.

All other assisted vaginal deliveries have a higher risk of failure and should be considered as a 'trial', which means they should be attempted in a place where immediate conversion to caesarean section can be undertaken. Also, presence of staff with expertise in AVB is essential.

Factors that may increase the risk of failure of AVB include:[3,4]

- maternal BMI greater than 30
- short maternal stature
- estimated fetal weight of greater than 4 kg or a clinically big baby
- head circumference above the 95th percentile
- occipito–posterior position
- station at mid-pelvis (above spines/spines+1) or when one-fifth of the head is palpable per abdomen

This list considers individual factors of concern, but each case requires judgement.

If the obstetrician considers that there is a high likelihood of success in the room, particularly with concern about fetal well-being then a transfer to theatre may cause more harm than good. Equally, one should not attempt a mid-cavity AVB in the room in situations where there is significant caput, moulding, and minimal or no descent with contractions.

Hence, clinical judgement should prevail over (high or low) confidence. It can be wiser to conduct a relatively easy delivery in theatre than to fail one in the room, without however reverting to theatre for every single case. An occupied theatre is not a reason to attempt a trial with a high chance of failure in the labour room; it is a reason to make expeditious efforts to open a second theatre.

## Appropriate Choice of Instrument – Ventouse versus Forceps

The clinical circumstances and the performing clinician's level of skill and confidence usually dictate the choice of the instrument.

Forceps and vacuum extraction are associated with different benefits and risks:

Vacuum extraction versus forceps assisted birth[3]

| More likely to fail at achieving vaginal birth | OR 1.7; 95% CI 1.3–2.2 |
| More likely to be associated with cephalhaematoma | OR 2.4; 95% CI 1.7–3.4 |
| More likely to be associated with maternal worries about baby | OR 2.2; 95% CI 1.2–3.9 |
| Less likely to be associated with significant maternal perineal and vaginal trauma | OR 0.4; 95% CI 0.3–0.5 |
| No more likely to be associated with delivery by caesarean birth* | OR 0.6; 95% CI 0.3–1.0 |
| No more likely to be associated with low 5-minute Apgar scores | OR 1.7; 95% CI 1.0–2.8 |
| No more likely to be associated with the need for phototherapy | OR 1.1; 95% CI 0.7–1.8 |

Adopted from RCOG Assisted Vaginal Birth (Green-Top Guideline No. 26).

*likely explanation is change of instrument to forceps

Forceps might be considered in preference, but not exclusively, for some accoucheurs in situations where there is significant caput (although it must be noted that the caput is on the leading aspect of the fetal head, whereas the flexion point is often posterior to this), and mainly in the case of poor/low maternal effort that cannot be corrected with coaching (for example, exhaustion or general anaesthesia). Individual chapters in this manual detail the factors associated with success and failure with each instrument, including technique and experience.

In situations where the woman or her family have objections to the method preferred clinically, the solution is neither to brush aside their fears nor to use an instrument likely to fail; the solution is an efficient evidence-based discussion of concerns and risks as described previously.

## Correct Use of Instrument

Confidence in performing spontaneous vaginal deliveries, theoretical knowledge, simulation training and clinical training under supervision are the pillars of AVB practice.

Accoucheurs leave on women and their birth partners memorable impressions including during AVB. Excessive force, inappropriate movement (including the infamous 'foot/knee on the bed' for counter-traction) and rocking the handle of the instrument up and down must be avoided at all times. It is important and possible to make it 'look beautiful' – use of fingers to apply, rotate and/or hold instruments, confirming their application discreetly (for example, checking that forceps match and lock on a side table and not on the woman's abdomen), and not with audible and visible uncertainty.

AVB should be performed by, or in the presence of, a clinician who has the knowledge, skills and experience necessary to assess the woman, complete the procedure, and manage any complications that arise, with the control and grace that is appropriate to the circumstances. Safety and elegance are not opposites, and speed comes with practice not with excessive haste.

It is crucial to document and explain any deviations and additional steps:

- Elective use of ventouse for rotation and descent and then conversion to forceps lift-out delivery
- If forceps were reapplied, when did this happen (before or after pulls), and what was the reason?

- If the ventouse cup was detached and reapplied, what was considered the likely reason?

- If an instrument was changed (for example Kielland's to Neville-Barnes or other direct traction forceps), when and why?


## Timely Recognition of Possible Complications and When to Abandon the Procedure

RCOG Assisted Vaginal Birth Green-Top Guideline No. 26 recommendations should be followed:

- Discontinue vacuum-assisted birth where there is no evidence of progressive descent with moderate traction during each pull of a correctly applied instrument by an experienced operator. If there is minimal descent with the first one or two pulls of a vacuum, the operator should consider whether the application is suboptimal, the fetal position has been incorrectly diagnosed or there is cephalopelvic disproportion. Less experienced operators should stop and seek a second opinion. Experienced operators should re-evaluate the clinical findings and either change approach or discontinue the procedure.

- Complete vacuum-assisted birth in the majority of cases with a maximum of three pulls to bring the fetal head on to the perineum. Three additional gentle pulls can be used to ease the head out of the perineum.

- Discontinue vacuum-assisted birth if there have been two 'pop-offs' of the instrument. Less experienced operators should seek senior support after one 'pop-off' to ensure the woman has the best chance of a successful assisted vaginal birth.

- Reconsider forceps if birth has not been achieved after three pulls. Unless vaginal birth is 'inevitable', conversion to caesarean section should be considered.

- Discontinue attempted forceps birth where the forceps cannot be applied easily, the handles do not approximate easily or if there is a lack of progressive descent with moderate traction.

- Discontinue rotational forceps birth if rotation is not easily achieved with gentle pressure.

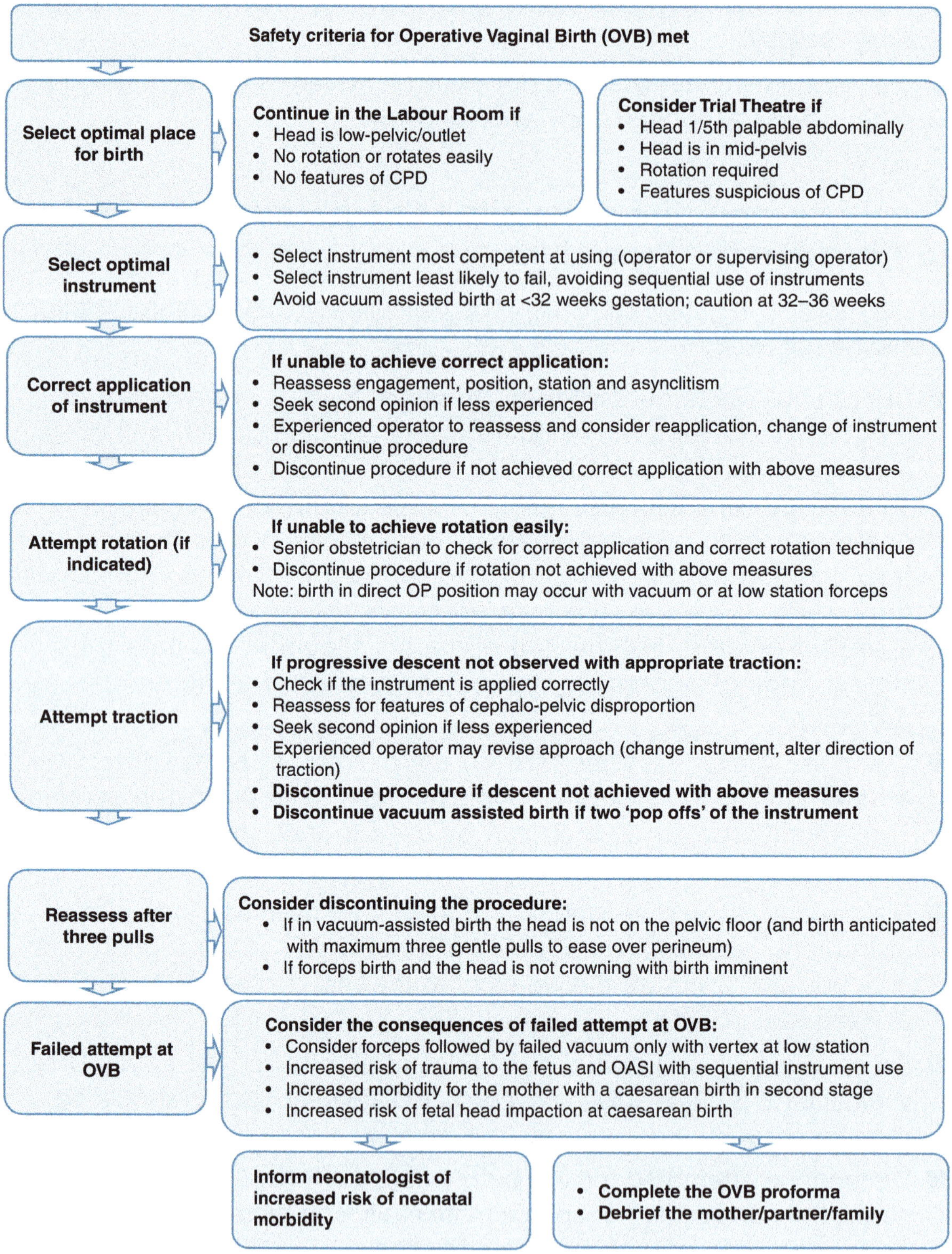

Safety criteria for Operative Vaginal Birth (OVB) met

**Select optimal place for birth**

**Continue in the Labour Room if**
- Head is low-pelvic/outlet
- No rotation or rotates easily
- No features of CPD

**Consider Trial Theatre if**
- Head 1/5th palpable abdominally
- Head is in mid-pelvis
- Rotation required
- Features suspicious of CPD

**Select optimal instrument**
- Select instrument most competent at using (operator or supervising operator)
- Select instrument least likely to fail, avoiding sequential use of instruments
- Avoid vacuum assisted birth at <32 weeks gestation; caution at 32–36 weeks

**Correct application of instrument**

**If unable to achieve correct application:**
- Reassess engagement, position, station and asynclitism
- Seek second opinion if less experienced
- Experienced operator to reassess and consider reapplication, change of instrument or discontinue procedure
- Discontinue procedure if not achieved correct application with above measures

**Attempt rotation (if indicated)**

**If unable to achieve rotation easily:**
- Senior obstetrician to check for correct application and correct rotation technique
- Discontinue procedure if rotation not achieved with above measures
Note: birth in direct OP position may occur with vacuum or at low station forceps

**Attempt traction**

**If progressive descent not observed with appropriate traction:**
- Check if the instrument is applied correctly
- Reassess for features of cephalo-pelvic disproportion
- Seek second opinion if less experienced
- Experienced operator may revise approach (change instrument, alter direction of traction)
- **Discontinue procedure if descent not achieved with above measures**
- **Discontinue vacuum assisted birth if two 'pop offs' of the instrument**

**Reassess after three pulls**

**Consider discontinuing the procedure:**
- If in vacuum-assisted birth the head is not on the pelvic floor (and birth anticipated with maximum three gentle pulls to ease over perineum)
- If forceps birth and the head is not crowning with birth imminent

**Failed attempt at OVB**

**Consider the consequences of failed attempt at OVB:**
- Consider forceps followed by failed vacuum only with vertex at low station
- Increased risk of trauma to the fetus and OASI with sequential instrument use
- Increased morbidity for the mother with a caesarean birth in second stage
- Increased risk of fetal head impaction at caesarean birth

Inform neonatologist of increased risk of neonatal morbidity

- **Complete the OVB proforma**
- **Debrief the mother/partner/family**

**Figure 8.2** The process of assisted vaginal birth.
Adopted from RCOG Assisted Vaginal Birth (Green-Top Guideline No. 26).

## Good Communication Throughout

Shared decision-making, good communication, and positive continuous support during labour and birth have the potential to reduce psychological morbidity following birth.[3]

Often what is needed is a couple of well-timed sentences explaining events as they occur. It is not realistic to expect a long, detailed explanation of shoulder dystocia, should it occur after AVB to a woman at low risk. It is equally unreasonable to manage it with a single sentence, for example that 'the baby's shoulders are stuck' and staff have to perform some quick and possibly uncomfortable manoeuvres to release them safely.

## Accurate Documentation

Documentation for assisted vaginal birth should include:

- Information provided to the woman before the procedure about risks and benefits
- Detailed assessment information (CTG, abdominal examination, vaginal examination)
- Decision time, indication, consent and detailed procedure description, including adverse outcomes (subsequent instruments, assisted vaginal birth failure, major obstetric haemorrhage, OASI, shoulder dystocia and significant neonatal complications)
- Plan for postnatal care
- Counselling in relation to subsequent pregnancies
- Paired cord blood samples result

Use of a standardised proforma (RCOG) is recommended.[3]

## Duty of Candour

**It is a professional responsibility to be honest with patients when things go wrong.**[3]

Duty of candour is not a tick-box exercise. It is the opportunity to explain what happened (even if the suboptimal outcome might be due to 'misadventure' in the presence of reasonable care), offer a sincere apology to the woman and her family for the adverse event with reassurance that measures will be put in place, including detailed review, development of solutions if any problems discovered, including learning & (re)training, and measures to prevent the same events recurring in the future, even if they were accidental.

## Follow-Up and Support

Ideally, the obstetrician who performed the AVB should review the woman before discharge home and offer her and her birth partner another discussion of events before, during and after the procedure, including possible complications and consequences for the future. This will allow them to understand the events and address all their concerns.

For women with persistent post-traumatic stress disorder (PTSD) symptoms, follow-up after one month with specialised professionals should be organised.[3]

Postnatal debriefing does not replace, it completes advanced planning and discussion (with use of translators where needed), and good communication during the events.

# Conclusion

The most effective way to minimise the ongoing human cost to both patients and staff, and the financial cost to the healthcare service, is to continue to improve safety in AVB, including regular practice using simulation, proactive risk management, parent-centred consent, appropriate supervision, good communication and comprehensive documentation.

# References

1.  NHS Litigation Authority. Ten Years of Maternity Claims, An Analysis of NHS Litigation Authority Data, ISBN: 978–0–9565019–2–9, 2012.

2.  Murphy DJ . Medico-legal considerations and operative vaginal delivery. Best Practice & Research Clinical Obstetrics & Gynaecology, Volume 56, 2019;114–24.

3.  RCOG. Assisted Vaginal Birth Green-Top Guideline No26, April 2020.

4.  NICE. Intrapartum Care CG190, 2017.

5.  Reitter A, Daviss B-A, Bisits A et al. Does pregnancy and/or shifting positions create more room in a woman's pelvis? Am J Obstet Gynecol 2014;211:662.e1-9.

6.  GMC Guidance: Decision making and consent, September 2020.

7.  RCOG. Consent and the Montgomery ruling, 2023. www.rcog.org.uk

8.  RCOG. Obtaining Valid Consent, Clinical Governance Advice No. 6, January 2015.

9.  RCOG. Consent Advice No. 11: Operative Vaginal Delivery, July 2010.

10. Murphy DJ, Liebling RE, Verity L, Swingler R, Patel R. Early maternal and neonatal morbidity associated with operative delivery in the second stage of labour: a cohort study. Lancet 2001;358:1203–7.

# Chapter 9
# Analgesia and Anaesthesia for Assisted Vaginal Birth

Rowena Pykett, George Bugg and David Levy

---

## Key Learning Points

- There are several techniques available to provide anaesthesia and analgesia for assisted vaginal birth (AVB), each with benefits and drawbacks dependent on the situation.

- An understanding of these techniques, in parallel with clinical assessment of the woman and scenario, will allow individualisation in each case.

---

This chapter deals with methods of analgesia and anaesthesia for AVB. Previous chapters have discussed the decision-making processes underpinning which type of birth is required and where to perform it; this chapter details the various types of analgesia and anaesthesia used in different situations.

AVB can be undertaken either in the labour room or in theatre. Estimation of the likelihood of vaginal birth proving successful is pivotal to informing decision-making in terms of analgesic and anaesthetic requirements.

Assessment of the woman by an experienced obstetrician will determine whether a birth can be conducted safely in the labour room. If there is a material risk of failed assisted vaginal birth requiring conversion to caesarean section, transfer to the operating theatre will be indicated.

The following points interact to influence the timing, location and instrument choice:

- efficacy of maternal effort and degree of descent with pushing
- station and position of the fetal head
- suspected fetal condition based on cardiotocography (CTG) monitoring and/or fetal blood sampling (FBS)
- analgesic requirements of the mother
- experience and confidence of the person conducting the birth.

# Local Anaesthetic Infiltration

The use of local anaesthesia for low cavity and outlet AVB, where it is expected to be straightforward, can allow the procedure to be carried out in the labour suite.

The operator must be confident that the birth can be achieved without recourse to caesarean section. Based on the woman's rapport with both midwife and obstetrician and her tolerance of vaginal examinations, an estimation can be made of her likely analgesic requirement and whether she is likely to tolerate an assisted vaginal birth under local anaesthesia alone.

Local anaesthesia has the advantages of wide availability and low cost. It is administered by the obstetrician attending the woman – an anaesthetist does not need to be available at the time. A local anaesthetic block will only relieve vaginal and perineal pain – there is no effect on the pain of uterine contractions.

## Local Anaesthetic Pharmacology

Local anaesthetics are reversible membrane-stabilising drugs; they block the sodium channels in the nerve membrane, preventing depolarisation and transmission of nerve impulses. A number of local anaesthetic agents are available: lidocaine is the most widely used in obstetrics in the UK. Various local anaesthetic preparations have been investigated. A recent Cochrane review has concluded that there is little difference between them.[1]

Lidocaine administered by infiltration has an onset of 5–10 minutes and duration of around 45 minutes.[2] There is no demonstrable benefit in adding adrenaline to local anaesthesia for pudendal infiltration – adrenaline-containing solutions are not routinely used in the UK.[3] Bupivacaine should not be used on account of its potential for systemic toxicity.

Lidocaine 1% contains 10 mg lidocaine per 1 ml solution. The recommended maximum dose for infiltration is 3 mg/kg. For a 70 kg woman, a total of 210 mg is allowed, equivalent to a volume of 21 ml 1% lidocaine.

It is important that the *cumulative* dose of local anaesthetic administered by all routes (including epidural) informs the calculation of the appropriate dose for an additional injection by the obstetrician. This is particularly important in a woman of low body mass, with whom it is easier to exceed a threshold total dose.

## Local Anaesthetic Toxicity

Systemic toxicity can develop secondary to either direct accidental administration into an artery or vein, or systemic absorption via vascular tissues of an excessive administered dose. Toxicity affects primarily the central nervous and cardiovascular systems (Table 9.1).

It is important to maintain verbal communication with the woman to discern symptoms while injecting local anaesthetic. Treatment of toxicity follows the general ABC principles of resuscitation with concurrent relief of aortocaval compression from the gravid uterus. Specific treatment for local anaesthetic-induced seizures or impending cardiac arrest is with Intralipid™ 20%. All labour wards should have an emergency box or trolley containing a LipidRescue™ box with instructions and equipment for infusion while resuscitation continues.[4]

## Pudendal Block and Perineal Infiltration

The majority of the innervation of the lower vagina, vulva and perineum is derived from the pudendal nerve (S2–4). The course of the nerve through the pelvis affords access for injection of local anaesthetic proximal to its division into terminal branches. The aim of blocking the pudendal nerve is to reduce sensation from the vagina and perineum sufficiently to allow low cavity and outlet AVB, including episiotomy and perineal repair.

**Table 9.1** Symptoms and signs of local anaesthetic toxicity

| Symptoms | Signs |
| --- | --- |
| Numbness of tongue or lips | Slurring of speech |
| Tinnitus | Drowsiness |
| Light-headedness | Convulsions |
| Anxiety | Cardiorespiratory arrest |

Although pudendal block has been used for many decades, there is little evidence of its anaesthetic effectiveness. Literature searches have failed to identify any research over the last 50 years demonstrating the efficacy of pudendal block for AVB.[5] Allowing adequate time for the local anaesthetic to work should provide better pain relief, providing the fetal condition permits.

There are two techniques, outlined below, for paravaginal pudendal block that are recommended and used commonly in the UK. There are variations in continental Europe where the pudendal nerve is reached through the perineal skin.

- Draw up 20 ml 1% lidocaine without adrenaline into a syringe.
- Attach a special guarded pudendal needle (Figure 9.1) the aim of which is to limit the depth of penetration of the needle and reduce the risk of needlestick injuries.
- Between contractions, palpate the left ischial spine with the left hand, hold the syringe with the right hand and guide the guarded needle between the index and middle finger of the left hand (irrespective of operator handedness).
- **Technique 1** – rest the index finger on the ischial spine and run the guarded needle between the fingers until it rests on the tissues 1 cm medial and posterior to the ischial spine (Figure 9.2).
- **Technique 2** – rest the middle finger on the ischial spine with the index finger above it, run the guarded needle between the fingers until it rests on the tissues 1 cm medial and anterior to the ischial spine (Figure 9.3).
- Unhook the needle guard and insert the needle 1 cm into the tissues adjacent to the anticipated course of the pudendal nerve.
- Large pudendal vessels run close to the nerve. It is particularly important to aspirate once the needle is in place. If blood is aspirated, re-site the needle.
- Inject 7 ml of anaesthetic, then guard the needle and withdraw.
- Repeat the procedure on the opposite side, changing the hand used to palpate the ischial spine and hold the syringe.

**Figure 9.1** Rocket™ pudendal needle.

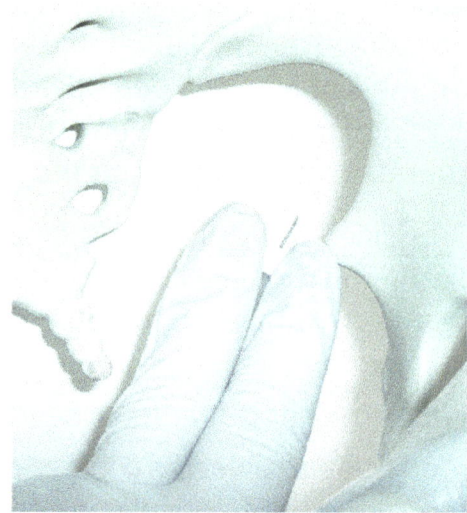

Figure 9.2 Technique 1 for paravaginal pudendal block.

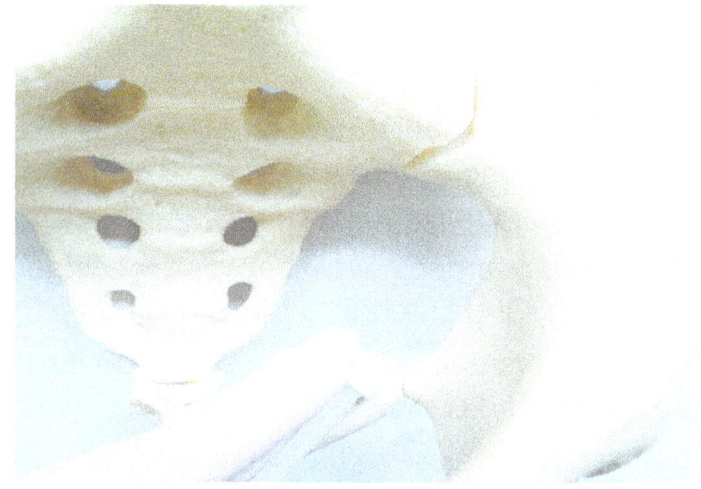

Figure 9.3 Technique 2 for paravaginal pudendal block.

■ Finally, inject the remaining 6 ml of local anaesthetic into the perineum in a radial pattern from the posterior fourchette, again remembering to aspirate before injection to avoid injecting anaesthetic directly into the bloodstream.

Occasionally the fetal head may be so low in the pelvis that palpating the ischial spines is impossible. In this scenario it would be unusual to require AVB. Perineal infiltration alone with 1% lidocaine 20 ml will permit adequate episiotomy. This method of perineal infiltration would also be appropriate for a birth requiring episiotomy alone.

While not universally performed, it is advisable to test the effectiveness of the block. This can be achieved by pinching the skin of the posterior fourchette with the operator's index finger and thumb. However, as the need for AVB is usually urgent, there is rarely time to rectify inadequate anaesthesia.

## Complications

Carried out as described, a pudendal block is generally a safe procedure with few complications. The risk of needlestick injury during this blind procedure should be minimised by gaining familiarity with the instrument. The potential exists for laceration from inadequate guarding of the needle and the formation of haematoma if the pudendal vessels are punctured. There are case reports of infection and abscess formation caused by inoculation of bacteria from the vagina. These conditions usually respond to conservative treatment with antibiotics. There is also potential for pudendal neuralgia if the nerve is traumatised, but no obstetric cases have been reported.

If there is any suspicion of accidental fetal injection, a neonatologist should be forewarned. Neonatal signs include hypotonia, seizures and cardiorespiratory compromise.[6]

# Regional Blockade

Neuraxial regional blockade is effected by injection of local anaesthetic and/or opioid into the epidural and/or subarachnoid spaces, blocking sensory nerves as they enter the spinal cord.

Epidural and spinal blocks are used on the labour ward for a number of reasons. Epidural analgesia is often used for pain relief (analgesia) during labour, with the advantage of the facility to provide *anaesthesia* for AVB in the room. Additionally, epidural top-up can be used for trial of AVB in theatre with the possibility of recourse to caesarean section (CS) if unsuccessful.

The sensory innervation of the uterus and cervix extends from T10 to L1; innervation of the vagina, vulva and perineum is derived from S2 to S4 nerve roots. Regional analgesia for labour or AVB requires block of sensation from these levels in order to provide adequate pain relief.

However, a dermatomal anaesthetic level to T4–5 is needed for adequate anaesthesia for CS – to block sensation from the abdominal peritoneum and viscera.

Single-shot spinal anaesthesia is generally not used for pain relief in labour on account of to its limited duration but has a vital role in providing anaesthesia for a trial of AVB in theatre.

When implementing a regional anaesthetic technique for AVB, there is a compromise to be made between impairment of the woman's ability to push (reduced muscle power) versus adequacy of CS anaesthesia if conversion is required. A forceps birth does not necessarily require any maternal effort, but the use of vacuum to assist birth usually requires co-ordination with maternal effort. There is a place for a less dense top-up of epidural anaesthesia for a vacuum birth with a caveat that further time will be required to provide anaesthesia for CS if vaginal birth proves unsuccessful.

Combined doses of local anaesthetic and opioid reduce the total quantity of each drug required to provide adequate analgesia (7). Table 9.2 compares epidural and spinal anaesthesia.

Provision of regional analgesia and anaesthesia requires the immediate availability of an experienced anaesthetist and should be available in UK consultant-led units. Contra-indications to regional analgesia are outlined in Table 9.3, and Table 9.4 outlines the complications.

**Table 9.2** Features and comparison of epidural and spinal anaesthetic

| Feature | Epidural |
| --- | --- |
| Onset of block | Up to 30 minutes |
| Duration of action | Can be extended |
| Efficacy of block | Possibly incomplete |
| Drug requirement | Large, risks systemic local anaesthetic toxicity |
| Technique | Infusion or repeated top-up |
| Headache | None unless accidental dural puncture |
| Hypotension | Uncommon |

**Table 9.3** Contra-indications to regional analgesia, with associated reasons

| Contra-indication | Reason |
| --- | --- |
| Refusal by woman | Subsequent legal claim |
| Lack of sufficient staff for continuous care | Delayed recognition of maternal or fetal compromise |
| Uncorrected anticoagulation or coagulopathy | Vertebral canal haematoma |
| Local or systemic sepsis | Vertebral canal abscess |
| Hypovolaemia or active haemorrhage | Cardiovascular collapse attributable to sympathetic blockade |

**Table 9.4** Complications of regional anaesthesia

| Risk | Event | Treatment |
|---|---|---|
| Accidental dural puncture | Accidental puncture of the meninges when siting epidural | Epidural blood patch (epidural injection of woman's own blood) best undertaken at 24–48 hours |
| | Leakage of cerebrospinal fluid can cause severe postural headache | Follow up until symptom-free |
| Total spinal | Large dose of local anaesthetic, intended for the epidural space, reaches the subarachnoid space | Emergency tracheal intubation and treatment of hypotension |
| | Block reaching cervical segments will impair diaphragmatic innervation | Caesarean birth of the baby, urgency dependent on fetal monitoring |
| Local anaesthetic toxicity | See 'local anaesthetic infiltration' | |

## Epidural Analgesia

Epidural analgesia is commonly provided in response to maternal request during the active first stage of labour. Alternatively, it may be jointly recommended by the anaesthetist and obstetrician anticipating a technically difficult anaesthetic in a woman at high risk of requiring AVB or caesarean section, for example an obese woman who has developed gestational diabetes with a high estimated fetal weight. Informed consent and disclosure of the material risks are essential. The UK Obstetric Anaesthetists' Association has prepared high-quality resources which the woman and her partner can access on a smartphone: https://www.labourpains.com/Information_Leaflets

An epidural is rarely used de novo for AVB unless an underlying maternal condition (e.g. severe aortic stenosis) contra-indicates the more rapid onset and profound sympathetic block of spinal anaesthesia.

Such women should be reviewed in an antenatal obstetric anaesthetic clinic where these challenges can be considered, and appropriate plans formulated.

Labour epidural analgesia is associated with an increased risk of AVB although the chance of caesarean section is not influenced.[8]

The following steps are undertaken:

- Discussion with woman and informed consent
- Fetal and maternal monitoring established
- Recent full blood count checked if necessary
- Secure IV access
- Aseptic technique – hat, mask, gown, handwashing, gloves, antiseptic preparation of woman's back, sterile drapes
- Epidural needle (Tuohy needle) and loss-of-resistance syringe assembled
- Interspinous spaces palpated
- Local anaesthetic injected into skin
- Epidural needle advanced through the skin, subcutaneous tissues and ligamentum flavum
- Aspirate syringe to exclude placement in blood vessel or subarachnoid space
- Epidural catheter threaded via needle into epidural space
- Catheter secured in place
- Loading dose of opioid and/or local anaesthetic, followed by continuous, programmed intermittent or patient-controlled boluses of the same drug mixture.

A bilateral block of cold sensation to T10 (just above the umbilicus) should relieve the pain of uterine contractions. A block above T6 should prompt cessation of the epidural infusion until the block regresses to T10.

When use of an existing labour epidural is planned for trial of AVB, the block must be sufficient to allow recourse to immediate caesarean section if vaginal birth proves unsuccessful. Once a decision is made for trial of AVB, the anaesthetist should be informed immediately in order that epidural top-up can be expedited. Conversion of labour epidural analgesia to surgical anaesthesia takes 15–20 minutes. Beginning the top-up in the labour room before transfer to theatre has the advantage of reducing the time to achieve surgical anaesthesia, but incurs the risks associated with minimal physiological monitoring during transfer to the operating theatre, for example hypotension and fetal compromise.

## Single-Shot Spinal Anaesthesia

In contrast to a large-gauge epidural needle (which facilitates passage of an epidural catheter), a finer gauge, tapered spinal needle is used for meningeal puncture and direct injection into the cerebrospinal fluid (CSF). Hyperbaric (denser than CSF) bupivacaine is used and the dose varied according to maternal body mass index and gestation. The addition of opioids can reduce the incidence of visceral pain.

Spinal anaesthesia is used for a trial of AVB in theatre where there is no or inadequate pre-existing epidural analgesia and there is a chance of recourse to caesarean section.

The block afforded by single-shot spinal anaesthesia develops faster than an epidural top-up. Surgical anaesthesia is achieved in 5–10 minutes. However, it can cause a sudden fall in blood pressure, with the potential for diminution of uteroplacental perfusion. Care must always be taken to minimise aortocaval compression by left-lateral tilt. The obstetrician must be mindful of the potential requirement for a quick birth if there is evidence of fetal compromise, and they should not leave theatre after institution of spinal anaesthesia.

The obstetrician must bear in mind that surgical anaesthesia is generally limited to 90 minutes, and that there is no facility to prolong the anaesthetic block. Caesarean section following unsuccessful AVB carries an increased risk of complications, especially postpartum haemorrhage. There should be good communication throughout between surgeon and anaesthetist so that adequate adjuvant analgesia can be given to keep the woman comfortable, and an awareness that general anaesthesia may be required if there is uncontrolled blood loss or surgery becomes protracted.

## Combined Spinal-Epidural Techniques

Less commonly used, combined spinal-epidural (CSE) analgesia and anaesthesia have the advantages of a rapid onset of spinal block with the flexibility afforded by an epidural catheter. An initial dose of subarachnoid local anaesthetic and opioid can be supplemented by further doses of drugs via the epidural catheter.

Such a technique could be useful if a surgical birth were anticipated to be complicated, for instance an elective caesarean section after multiple previous abdominal surgeries.

# General Anaesthesia

General anaesthesia may be required if an unsuccessful AVB necessitates caesarean section and the regional block is inadequate. A much less common scenario would be where an AVB under local anaesthesia was thought to be possible but has been unsuccessful, and regional anaesthesia was absolutely contra-indicated for any reason.

This is usually a tense situation for all involved, and good communication is vital. The safety of the mother is of utmost importance; time and patience are vital for a safe general anaesthetic even when there are significant fetal concerns.

The main maternal risks of general anaesthesia are airway problems such as failed intubation, aspiration of gastric contents and anaphylaxis to the neuromuscular blocking drug succinylcholine. General anaesthetic drugs are innocuous to the fetus in the long term although transient respiratory depression, requirement for active resuscitation and low Apgar scores are more common after general anaesthesia compared with regional blockade, regardless of events prior to caesarean section.

# Concerns Following Birth

When a birth has been performed under regional anaesthesia, it is easy to neglect subsequent postpartum analgesia as the woman will be comfortable at the time of birth. It is common to give diclofenac per rectum following AVB (provided there are no contra-indications), and to prescribe regular analgesia as appropriate for the following days.

Venous thromboembolism (VTE) has been highlighted as a leading cause of maternal mortality in successive triennial mortality reports and must be considered following AVB. Proformas for scoring women's individual risk factors are used. The increased risk of VTE following mid-cavity AVB versus low cavity birth is reflected by an increased score.[9]

# References

1.  Novikova N, Cluver C. Local anaesthetic nerve block for pain management in labour. Cochrane Db Syst Rev. 2012;(4):CD009200.

2.  Palmer C, D'Angelo R, Peach M. *Obstetric Anaesthesia*. Oxford, UK: Oxford University Press; 2011. p.440.

3.  Schierup L, Schmidt JF, Jensen AT, Rye BAO. Pudendal block in vaginal deliveries mepivacaine with and without epinephrine. Acta Obstet Gyn Scan. 1988;67(3):195–7.

4.  LipidRescue [Internet]. [cited 14 Jan 2022]. http://lipidrescue.org/

5.  Scudamore JH, Yates MJ. Pudendal block – a misnomer? Lancet. 1966;287(7427):23–4.

6.  Sinclair JC, Fox HA, Lentz JF, Fuld GL, Murphy J. Intoxication of the fetus by a local anesthetic – a newly recognized complication of maternal caudal anesthesia. New Engl J Medicine. 1965;273 (22):1173–7.

7.  Chestnut D, Wong C, Tsen L et al. *Chestnut's Obstetric Anesthesia: Principles and Practice*. 6th ed. New York: Elsevier; 2019. p. 1382.

8.  Murphy DJ, Strachan BK, Bahl R, on behalf of the Royal College of Obstetricians and Gynaecologists. Assisted Vaginal Birth: Green-Top Guideline No. 26. Bjog Int J Obstetrics Gynaecol. 2020; 127: e70–e112.

9.  Nelson-Piercy C, McCallum P, Mackillop L. Thrombosis and Embolism during Pregnancy and the Puerperium, Reducing the Risk (Green-Top Guideline No. 37a). Royal College of Obstetricians and Gynaecologists; 2015.

# Index

*Please note:* page numbers in *italic type* indicate illustrations or tables

For EU product safety concerns, contact us at Calle de José Abascal, 56–1°, 28003 Madrid, Spain or eugpsr@cambridge.org.

www.ingramcontent.com/pod-product-compliance
Ingram Content Group UK Ltd.
Pitfield, Milton Keynes, MK11 3LW, UK
UKHW050012071225
465726UK00008B/285